# Health

## personal & communal

# Health
## personal & communal

**John Gibson** MD, FRCPSYCH, DPM
*with illustrations by* Audrey Besterman

Faber & Faber
3 Queen Square London

First published in 1959
by Faber and Faber Limited
3 Queen Square London WC1
Second edition 1963
First published in this edition 1963
Reprinted 1966
Third edition 1968
Reprinted 1971 and 1973
Fourth edition 1976
Printed in Great Britain by
Butler & Tanner Ltd, Frome and London
All rights reserved

© *John Gibson*
*1959*

ISBN 0 571 04909 5 (*Faber Paperbacks*)
ISBN 0 571 04908 7 (*hard-bound edition*)

## Preface to the Fourth Edition

For the fourth edition this book has been completely revised. The re-organization of the National Health service is described. A new chapter has been added on the dangers to health from alcohol, smoking and drugs, and among the other new material are sections on Occupational Health Services, Australian antigen, Pharaoh's ants, the Health and Safety at Work Act, and the Chronically Sick and Disabled Persons Act.

J.G.

*June 1976*

## Acknowledgements

For information and advice I am much indebted to: Dr. P. Alexander, Chester Beatty Research Institute (Radiation Risks); C. S. Miles, Esq., United Dairies Ltd. (Milk); the Royal Society for the Prevention of Accidents (Accidents in the Home); and S. L. Wedge, Esq., Department of Employment and Productivity, Caterham.

I would also like to thank the British Red Cross Society, who have allowed me to use two of the drawings from their book, *Practical Aids for the Disabled*.

# Contents

# Illustrations

# Chapter One

# HEALTH FOR EVERYONE

Hygiene is the science of health. The word comes from the name of a Greek goddess, Hygeia, the daughter of the first god-physician, Aesculapius, and describes all the activities that produce a healthy body and mind and prevent disease.

Some of these activities are personal habits of one's own (such as the kind of food one eats and how much sleep one takes); some are family activities (such as living together in a house); some are the result of the work for the larger community in which one lives (such as the supply of water and the disposal of sewage); some are national activities (such as a Health Service); and some are international activities settled by agreement among nations (such as the precautions taken to prevent the spread of disease from one country to another).

The ways in which health can be promoted and disease prevented are described in this book. When a nurse comes to this part of her studies she has to consider not how sick people are nursed, but how they are prevented from becoming ill. She will see that many of the subjects of this study are undertakings such as growing enough of the right sorts of food, providing clean milk and water, and building good houses, in achieving which people other than doctors and nurses are primarily employed: farmers in producing milk, meat and grain, water engineers in supplying water, town planners, architects and builders in erecting houses. As many of the communal activities and responsibilities must necessarily be established by law, the nurse should consider how she is governed and know something of the health services provided by the local government of the place in which she lives and by the government of the country, services that guard everyone in health and disease. She should also know something of the voluntary societies and organizations to which sick or handicapped people or their relatives or anyone interested can turn for help and advice.

## The British Health Services

The British Health Services are organized at four levels:

1. The Department of Health and Social Security
2. Regional Health Authorities
3. Area Health Authorities
4. Districts.

**The Department of Health and Social Security.** This department is the central government department (with its principal offices in London) concerned with the health of the nation and the social security provisions for the people. In Wales the *Welsh Office* (in Cardiff) is the responsible department, in Scotland the *Scottish Home and Health Department* (in Edinburgh), and in Northern Ireland (in Belfast) the *Department of Health and Social Service.*

The Secretary of State for Health and Social Security in England and Wales determines national policies and priorities and is responsible to Parliament for the service as a whole. The running of the service is delegated by the Department to the Regional Health Authorities and through them to the Area Health Authorities.

**Regional Health Authorities.** There are fourteen Regional Health Authorities in England. Because of their smaller size, Wales and Scotland do not have Regional Health Authorities, the running of the service in these countries being delegated directly to the Area Health Authorities from the Welsh Office in Wales and the Scottish Home and Health Department in Scotland.

In England the Regional Health Authorities are responsible for:

(a) regional planning of the health service and the allocation of resources,

(b) those services that are best organized regionally, e.g. the siting, planning and design of large hospitals,

(c) checking the performance of their Area Health Authorities against agreed plans.

**Area Health Authorities.** There are ninety Area Health Authorities in England, eight in Wales and fifteen in Scotland. In Northern

Ireland four *Health and Social Services Boards* are responsible for both health and personal social services. Arrangements in London are slightly different from those in the rest of England because it has a large number of teaching hospitals (a teaching hospital, in this sense, is one in which medical students are taught) and because it has a different local government structure. The Area Health Authorities usually have the same geographical boundaries as the Local Government Authorities (in some places one Area Health Authority serves two or three Local Government Authorities) or the London Boroughs. This enables co-ordination to take place between the principal departments concerned: health services, social services and education.

The principal work of an Area Health Authority is:

(a) the organization of the family practitioner service and its integration with other parts of the health service,

(b) the organization and running of hospitals,

(c) the provision of dental, pharmaceutical and ophthalmic services,

(d) the provision of *community health services*, including: school health service, home (district) nursing, ambulance service, health centres, clinics for mothers and young children, family planning, immunization, old people, etc., supervision of private nursing homes, health education in schools and the community, cooperation with voluntary organizations.

**Districts** are the smallest sections in the health service. A District serves on an average 250,000 people and has in it at least one general hospital. Services in it are organized by a *District Management Team* of senior staff—a consultant, a general practitioner, a community physician, a nurse, an administrator and a treasurer.

**Community Health Councils** represent the interests of the public in its own local health services. There is usually one Council for each part of an area which forms a natural health district, e.g. one determined by geographical conditions, bus and railway services, hospital siting, local wishes and traditions. The members of a Council are chosen partly by local authorities, partly by local voluntary organizations, partly by other local organizations and some members are appointed by the Regional Health Authority. The Area Health Authority is expected to consult the Council, as representing the public for whom the service exists, about any plans it may have for development of the service and any important variations which would affect the public.

**Health Service Commissioner.** The Health Service Commissioner (or 'Ombudsman' as he is called, the name being taken from that of a similar office in Sweden) considers certain kinds of complaints about the health services.

**Other Government Departments.** The *Department of the Environment* is concerned with land use planning, road building and traffic management, water supplies and sewerage, among other duties.

The *Ministry of Agriculture, Fisheries and Food* is concerned in the provision of food and the prevention of disease in farm animals.

The *Department of Education and Science* is concerned in educational provisions for children including those who are blind, partially sighted, or handicapped in other ways. The *Department of Employment* is concerned in the health of factory workers, industrial rehabilitation of injured or sick workpeople, and the training and employment of the blind.

The *Home Office* is concerned in the care of the 'deprived child' (in this context, a healthy, normal child who has no home) and in the control of dangerous drugs.

Certain statutory bodies are established by Parliament: the *General Medical Council* for the training of medical students and the registration of doctors; the *General Nursing Council* for the training and registration of nurses; and the *Central Midwives' Board* for the training, enrolment and supervision of midwives.

**National Insurance and Supplementary Allowances.** People in Britain are insured under the *National Insurance Act, 1946*. This is a compulsory insurance scheme, in which in return for weekly contributions a person is entitled to financial benefits in certain circumstances. The Act is a complicated one for it has to consider all classes of people, those who are employed by someone else and are paid a wage or salary, those who are self-employed, and those who are not gainfully employed. Those who are employed by someone else have a part of the weekly contribution paid by the employer. Contributions are payable in National Insurance Stamps.

The benefits provided under the scheme include:

(a) a Sickness Benefit during illness;
(b) an Unemployment Benefit during unemployment;
(c) a Maternity Benefit and a Grant of money on the birth of a child;
(d) a Retirement Benefit after retirement from work;
(e) a Widow's Pension;
(f) a Death Grant.

The *National Insurance Act, 1959,* introduced into National Insurance a scheme of graduated contributions (discontinued in April 1975) and retirement pensions related to employees' earnings; contributions are paid by both employer and employee. Employees covered by a recognized superannuation scheme or occupational pension scheme could be contracted out of this graduated part of the National Insurance scheme, provided that certain conditions were satisfied. The *National Insurance Act, 1966,* introduced into National Insurance a system of earnings-related payments in addition to the ordinary sickness, industrial injury, maternity allowances and unemployment benefits.

By these measures it is hoped that a person will not become gravely impoverished by sickness, unemployment or old age.

*Industrial Benefits* are payable if a workman is injured or killed at work or suffers from certain specified diseases arising out of his work (e.g. silicosis in miners).

Under the *Family Allowances Act* the mother of two or more children can claim a weekly sum, which it is intended she should spend on the family as a whole. In certain circumstances (for instance, if the mother has died or does not look after her children) the money is payable to the father. In one-parent families the money is paid for the first child as well as for any other children since 1976. Low income families can also be helped by *Family Income Supplement*.

Under the *Social Security Acts* a state scheme provides financial assistance to necessitous people, and the Local Authority has a duty to provide residential accommodation for the old, the infirm, the homeless and the disabled, and welfare services for the blind, the deaf and dumb, and other crippled people. Over two million people a year apply for assistance. They are usually old people, people long unemployed or for other reasons not entitled to benefit under the national insurance schemes, unmarried mothers, deserted wives, wives and children of men in prison, blind people. Assistance is usually in the form of money to pay for rent, food, heating and other necessities of life. Difficulties are encountered in dealing with the chronic unemployed, vagrants, and 'problem families' whose members are socially incapable and often mentally and physically handicapped.

**Societies and Organizations.** Many societies and organizations exist for the promotion of hygiene, the alleviation of disease, the promotion of research, and the education of the public in health matters. Among them are:

*The Royal Society of Health*, 13 Grosvenor Place, London SW1X 1EN, which is interested in all aspects of communal health, at home and abroad, and conducts examinations in hygiene and sanitation.

*The Queen's Nursing Institute*, 57 Lower Belgrave Street, London, S.W.1., which provides training in district nursing and midwifery.

*Family Welfare Association Ltd.*, 501–5 Kingsland Road, London E8 4AU, which publishes a register of charities and a guide to the social services of the country, provides advice and guidance in personal and family problems, conducts research into social problems, etc.

*National Association for Maternity and Child Welfare*, Tavistock House North, Tavistock Square, London, W.C.1., promotes the welfare of mothers and children by conferences, publications and research.

*The Chest and Heart Association*, Tavistock House North, Tavistock Square, London, W.C.1., conducts research, education and propaganda in the field of tuberculosis and diseases of the chest and heart.

*National Association for Mental Health*, 39 Queen Anne Street, London, W.1., has for its object the promotion of mental health, publishes books and pamphlets, conducts training courses, etc.

*National Society for Mentally Handicapped Children*, 86 Newman Street, London, W.1., promotes research into mental disorders and mental retardation, and has many local societies affiliated to it.

*Royal Society for the Prevention of Accidents*, Cannon House, Priory Queensway, Birmingham B1 6BS, aims at the prevention of accidents of all kinds.

The Family Welfare Association publishes further information about these societies and many others in its 'Annual Charities Register'. The same association publishes annually a 'Guide to the Social Services' of Britain, in which will be found details of National Insurance, Social Security, etc., and of the rates of contributions, benefits, pensions, etc.

# Chapter Two

# PERSONAL HEALTH

The services of a country, provided nationally or locally, protect everybody's health in many ways; but each individual is left to apply to himself, and to those he is responsible for, certain principles of personal hygiene. In these he is allowed much choice. But it is important that in making his choice he should be well informed, and a nurse should know what advice to give her patients on such personal matters affecting health as eating, drinking and smoking; work, rest, exercise and sleep; personal cleanliness; and clothing.

**Eating and Drinking.** Meals should be regular, of varied content and appetizing. Details of adequate diets are given in the next chapter. An adequate diet should provide adequate calories, proteins, fats, carbohydrates, vitamins, minerals and water; it should be able to supply sufficient energy to the body, to build up the tissues of a growing child, and to replace worn-out tissues. The ordinary mixed meals of an average British household are usually adequate for all these purposes, and only rarely is malnutrition seen. In the home special attention has to be paid to the diet of children, expectant mothers and breast-feeding mothers, who require a diet rich in protein and of a high energy value. Appetite is usually an excellent guide; but where food is plentiful, over-eating is likely to occur and may lead to dangerous obesity.

**Work.** The amount and kinds of work that people do vary very much. Work must be:

within the physical capacity of the individual;

and should be both:

suitable for his intelligence and temperament, and

emotionally satisfying.

As people vary in physique, intelligence and temperament, so may they vary in their choice of work. Some like regular work with regular hours and little change, and are content with an office desk or a factory bench; some like work that varies in amount and intensity and that changes frequently. Some find responsibility and leadership stimulating, make decisions easily, and can direct others; some may prefer to be directed and are good at carrying out work that they cannot initiate. Either type may develop nervous symptoms if they find themselves in the wrong job.

**Exercise and Games.** Some form of physical exercise is necessary if positive health is to be achieved and maintained, and people who do not get it in their work should take it in games or exercise. Physical exercise promotes health in many ways: it maintains the circulatory system in a state of efficiency, ventilates the lungs, promotes digestion, keeps the skin clean by perspiration, and maintains the efficiency of the voluntary muscles and the nervous system. The heart learns to achieve what is demanded of it with the minimum of effort so that the pulse rate is kept as low as possible and the blood pressure is not unduly raised; nervous responses are made more quickly; the voluntary muscles have an increased tone and size; the amount of fat in the body is kept at a healthy level. The physically fit man can be identified by his erect posture, his taut abdominal musculature, his clear skin, and his mental alertness.

At school, eurhythmics, gymnastics and games are organized as part of the scheme of physical education. After a person has left school, the amount of exercise taken will largely depend upon his individual efforts, interest and skills. Walking, climbing, hiking, athletics, cycling, swimming, tennis, cricket, football, hockey, riding, golf, fishing and shooting have their particular appeal to different people, and many of them can, in diminishing amounts, be carried on with benefit into old age. Exercise in the open air is much more invigorating than exercise under cover, and some should be taken every day. There appears to be no risk in allowing a girl or woman to join in ordinary games during menstruation.

**Rest and Relaxation.** Most people on regular work benefit from short rest periods, in which drinks or snacks may be taken, during the day. Fatigue may be the result of too much hard work done in too short a space of time; of inadequate ventilation in the place of work; of unsuspected disease; or of boredom produced by monotonous work, inactivity or lack of adequate stimulation.

Tired or bored people may be tempted to take drugs.

Some people devote all their interest to their work and have little time or inclination for other activities. Many are all the better for a hobby or interest outside their work, especially those whose work is monotonous, uncreative or emotionally unsatisfying.

**Sleeping.** Young babies sleep nearly all day, older babies for most of the day. Children require from ten to twelve hours' sleep in every twenty-four hours. The amount that an adult requires shows individual variation of between five and nine hours a night. In their sleeping habits people may be divided into two classes: those who wake early and completely, are at their best in the morning, tire in the evening, and go to bed early; and those who are sleepy in the morning, improve as the day goes on, are at their best at night, and go to bed late. Many people are refreshed by a short nap of ten or fifteen minutes in the middle of the day or early evening.

A bedroom should be quiet, without glaring lights, and well ventilated. The bed should have sufficient bedclothes to keep a sleeper warm without making him hot. Some people, and especially young children, sleep quite well with very few bedclothes over them.

**Personal Cleanliness.** The skin is washed to remove dirt, dried perspiration, dead skin cells and micro-organisms, and to give the body a pleasant smell. Daily baths are necessary for nurses, for people with dirty work and during hot weather; otherwise a hot bath twice or three times a week is adequate. Taken before going to bed it may promote sleep. A daily cold bath is often recommended as a stimulant and health-promoting measure.

A shower bath is preferable to an ordinary bath for two reasons: (1) all dirt is washed off the body straight down the drain, and (2) it uses much less hot water and therefore reduces heating costs.

Washing the hands is very important. The hands should be washed after every visit to the lavatory, before preparing or eating food, before feeding children or others, and after changing babies.

The nails should be kept short by filing or cutting twice a week, should not be allowed to project beyond the tips of the fingers, and should be kept clean with a nailbrush. Wet and dry barrier creams may be used to protect the hands during wet and dirty work.

Feet that perspire easily should be washed daily, a daily change being made of socks and stockings. The spaces between the third and fourth and between the fourth and fifth toes should be inspected for evidence of ringworm infection, which commonly makes the skin there sodden, white and thickened.

A man's hair should be washed once a week or oftener if his occupation is a dirty one. A woman's hair should be kept clean and well groomed.

**Clothing.** Clothing is worn for three purposes: (1) to keep the body warm and conserve heat in cold weather, (2) as a protection from the sun, the wind and the rain, and (3) for personal adornment.

Clothes should be suitable for the work to be done in them and should not restrict movements or be too tight. Heat is conserved better by several layers of thin material than by one of thick because the air between the layers, air being a bad conductor of heat, prevents heat from leaving the body; and loose clothes are warmer than tight-fitting ones. Wet clothes are cold to the body because they are better conductors of heat than dry clothes and because the evaporation of water from them cools the body.

Clothes may be made of natural substances, such as wool, cotton and silk, or of man-made fibres, such as nylon and Terylene. Each has various advantages and disadvantages.

*Wool* has the advantages of feeling warm, of being light, and of not absorbing water easily. Wool irritates the skin of some people, and pure wool is expensive. Many 'new wool' garments are machine-washable, but care has to be taken in drying them because they are liable to go out of shape.

*Cotton* has the advantages of being cheap, of being washable and boilable, and of not shrinking as easily as wool. It has the disadvantages of absorbing water quickly and thereby feeling cold, and in some forms, especially flannelette and winceyette, of catching fire easily and burning quickly.

*Silk* has the advantages of not shrinking and of feeling cool in summer and warm in winter; it has the disadvantage of being too expensive for most people.

The new *man-made fibres* have the advantages of being strong and easily washed, of drying quickly, and of not being eaten by moths. They have the disadvantages of absorbing little moisture and of attracting dirt.

**Shoes.** Shoes are worn for three purposes: (1) support of the foot, (2) protection of the foot from injury, cold, wet and dirt, and (3) personal adornment.

Shoes are usually made of leather because leather is both strong and slightly yielding, able to stand up to the strains put upon it, and hard-wearing, and can both let air through and absorb moisture from the foot. Children's shoes often have soles made of resin-rubber, which is light, tough, flexible and harder wearing than leather. Rubber may be used for making waterproof soles and for boots that must be absolutely water-tight: it cannot 'breathe' like leather and so may make the feet hot and sweaty.

Men's shoes are almost invariably chosen for their fit, and being usually of the lace-up variety with low heels and rounded toecaps do not often cause foot trouble. They should be as light as possible for the work to be done in them.

Women's shoes are more likely to cause trouble because they are more often chosen for their appearance than their fit. Feet that have to stand on hard pavements and floors and do a lot of walking should be given adequate support below and above the insteps; the toes should be allowed plenty of room and not be cramped. For walking and standing a shoe should have a broad heel and be cut high at the front and sides. Too high a heel must be avoided because it throws the foot into the front of the shoe and cramps the toes. A woman should know her size and fit. Her fitting may be anywhere between AAA, the narrowest, and E, the broadest. She may have to try the products of several manufacturers before she finds the shoe most suited to her foot, and thereafter she should stick to that manufacturer. She should not buy shoes in a hurry, should try on both shoes, and should not buy a pair until she is quite satisfied about the fit.

Bedroom slippers should be worn only in the bedroom and bathroom, and as they give inadequate support to the feet they should not be used for walking about the house or working in it.

Children's shoes should be like men's—low-heeled, laced and with rounded toecaps, broad enough to take the toes comfortably. Well-made sandals may be worn for part of the day. Children's shoes should be changed as the foot grows. Ideally a new pair of shoes of the right size and shape should be bought when required; but as shoes are expensive and often not worn out by the time they are outgrown, it is a common practice to pass them down from one child to another, a practice in which there is no particular harm so long as the feet of the children concerned have the same sort of shape and the shoes are not distorted by wear. What is important is that a child should not have to wear shoes that are too small for him and might deform his feet or shoes that are too large. Plimsolls should be worn only for games and Wellingtons only out of doors in wet weather.

People who are on their feet all day should, if they can, change their shoes and stockings during the day. It is well to have a change of shoes so that the same pair is not worn for two days in succession; while the shoes are not being worn they will get rid of the moisture they have absorbed from the feet. Wet shoes should not be dried in front of a fire because heat makes leather hard.

# Chapter Three

# FOOD

Nutrition is one of the most important factors in the production and maintenance of health and the prevention of disease. It is essential that people should eat the right amount of the right kinds of food. What is the right amount depends upon the nutritional needs of an individual, which vary with age, sex, rate of growth, amount of work done, state of nutrition, state of health, and climate. The ordinary diet of people in this country usually provides an adequate amount of all the foodstuffs necessary for health and normal development, but ill people, poor people, old people and ignorant people may have a diet deficient in amount or in some essential constituent, and it is important for their physical and mental health that these deficiencies be rectified.

The three essential functions of food are:

1. To provide the necessary materials for the building up of the tissues of a growing child.

2. To provide the materials for the replacement of tissues worn out in normal activity or broken down by disease-processes, and to provide the materials from which are made the enzymes, hormones and other secretions from various tissues.

3. To provide a source of energy for the body.

The *essential foodstuffs* are:

1. *Proteins.* Proteins are necessary for the building and replacement of tissues, are part of the fundamental structure of cells, and are essential components of enzymes, hormones and other secretions. They are composed of carbon, hydrogen, and oxygen, of nitrogen (of which they are almost the only source), and of some of the minerals. They are composed of combinations of smaller structures called amino-acids. The usual sources of them in a diet are meat, fish, milk, eggs, poultry, beans and peas.

2. *Carbohydrates.* Carbohydrates are necessary as a source of energy. Being easily obtainable, cheap and easily digested they are

the major source of food. They are formed of carbon, hydrogen and oxygen in various proportions and occur as sugars and starches. The usual sources of them are sugar, bread, cereals, potatoes, honey, jam and dried fruit.

3. *Fats.* Fats are necessary to provide a store of fuel in the body, in which they are easily stored, and to provide the fat-soluble vitamins. Under the term fat are included the true fats, which are composed of fatty acids, the lipids, which are similar to the fats in structure, and the sterols, which are dissimilar in structure but related in function. The usual sources of the fats are milk, cream, margarine, lard, fat meat, and vegetable oils.

4. *Vitamins.* The vitamins are the essential food factors, chemical substances essential for normal growth and development, for building up resistance to bacterial infection, for the maintenance of nervous stability, for the normal functioning of the digestive tract, and for many other chemical activities in the body. Vitamins A and D are supplied in fatty food, especially fish-liver oils, milk, butter and vitaminized margarine. The vitamin B complex is supplied in whole-meal bread, lean meat, yeast, liver, kidneys and egg. Vitamin C is supplied in fresh fruit (oranges, lemons, grapefruit, tomatoes), in vegetables (spinach, parsley, cabbage, peas, potatoes, lettuce), and in blackcurrant juice and rose-hip juice; it is destroyed by cooking and when food is kept hot for a few hours. Vitamin E is supplied in vegetables, fruit and dairy produce. Vitamin K is supplied in green leaves, liver and egg-yolk.

5. *Minerals.* The minerals necessary for the body include calcium, phosphorus, sulphur, chlorine, iodine, sodium, magnesium, iron and copper. Some of them are necessary in minute quantities. All are essential for normal growth, cell life, or the regeneration of tissues. As they occur naturally in many kinds of food, they are provided in adequate amounts by normal diets.

6. *Water.* Water is essential for the life of all cells, is the medium in which many constituents of the body are held dissolved, forms the greater part of the various fluids secreted within the body, and regulates the temperature of the body. It is present in all natural foodstuffs and is also formed in the body by metabolic processes.

## Average Calorie Values of Common Helpings of Some Foods

| *Meats* | | kcal |
|---|---|---|
| Bacon: lean | 2 oz. | 175 |
| fat | 2 oz. | 260 |
| Beef: roast | 4 oz. | 210 |
| Ham: lean | 4 oz. | 265 |
| fat | 4 oz. | 375 |
| Lamb: lean | 4 oz. | 230 |
| fat | 4 oz. | 375 |
| Liver | 4 oz. | 160 |
| Mutton: lean | 4 oz. | 230 |
| fat | 4 oz. | 370 |
| Pork: lean | 4 oz. | 270 |
| fat | 4 oz. | 450 |
| Sausage: beef | 2 oz. | 120 |
| pork | 2 oz. | 145 |

| *Fish* | | |
|---|---|---|
| Cod, fillet | 4 oz. | 95 |
| Haddock: | | |
| fresh | 4 oz. | 115 |
| smoked | 4 oz. | 120 |
| Halibut | 4 oz. | 140 |
| Herring | one | 190 |
| Mackerel | 4 oz. | 90 |
| Salmon: fresh | 4 oz. | 155 |
| tinned | 4 oz. | 190 |
| Sardines | 2 oz. | 160 |
| Egg | one | 80 |

| *Fruits and Vegetables* | | kcal |
|---|---|---|
| Apple | one | 40 |
| Beans: baked | 4 oz. | 100 |
| broad | 2 oz. | 30 |
| runner | 4 oz. | 15 |
| Cauliflower | 4 oz. | 20 |
| Lettuce | 2 oz. | 10 |
| Prunes, dried | 2 oz. | 75 |
| Potatoes: | | |
| boiled | 4 oz. | 95 |
| fried | 4 oz. | 270 |

| *Mainly Carbohydrate Foods* | | kcal |
|---|---|---|
| Arrowroot | 1 oz. | 100 |
| Biscuits: plain | 1 oz. | 105 |
| sweet | 1 oz. | 135 |
| Bread | 1 oz. | 70 |
| Cake: plain | 2 oz. | 150 |
| rich | 2 oz. | 210 |
| Cornflakes | 1 oz. | 115 |
| Flour | 1 oz. | 100 |
| Honey | 1 oz. | 80 |
| Jam | 1 oz. | 70 |
| Oatmeal | 1 oz. | 110 |
| Rice, dry | 2 oz. | 180 |
| Sago | 2 oz. | 195 |
| Sugar, white | $\frac{1}{2}$ oz. | 55 |

| *Milk and Milk Products* | | |
|---|---|---|
| Butter | $\frac{1}{4}$ oz. | 65 |
| Cheese: Cheddar | 1 oz. | 120 |
| cream | 1 oz. | 155 |
| Dutch | 1 oz. | 90 |
| Margarine | $\frac{1}{4}$ oz. | 55 |
| Milk, whole | 1 glass | 200 |
| *Chocolate:* plain | 2 oz. | 300 |
| milk | 2 oz. | 300 |
| *Soup:* clear | 4 oz. | 20 |
| thick | 4 oz. | 65 |

| *Fruits and Vegetables* | | kcal |
|---|---|---|
| Banana | one | 50 |
| Brussels sprouts | 4 oz. | 20 |
| Cabbage | 4 oz. | 20 |
| Carrot | 2 oz. | 15 |
| Grapefruit | 4 oz. | 25 |
| Orange | one | 40 |
| Peaches, tinned | 4 oz. | 75 |
| Raspberries | 4 oz. | 25 |
| Strawberries | 4 oz. | 30 |

**Food as Energy.** Food has to provide energy for the body, and the value of food as a source of energy is expressed in calories or in joules. A kilocalorie is the amount of heat required to raise the temperature of a kilogram of water by 1° Centigrade. (The kilocalorie used in reckoning the heat-producing value of food is a thousand times larger than the calorie used in physics.)

Calories and joules are related in the following way: 1 calorie = 4·186 joules, or 1 kilocalorie (kcal) = 4·186 kilojoules (kJ).

The energy produced by carbohydrates, fat and protein when they are completely broken down in the body is:

Carbohydrates 4 kcal (16 kJ) per gram
Fat 9 kcal (38 kJ) per gram
Protein 4 kcal (17 kJ) per gram

The vitamins, minerals, and water in food do not supply any energy.

**Energy Requirements.** The number of kilocalories that people require per day in this country is:

### Children

| | |
|---|---|
| Under 1 year | 100–110 kcal per kg (45–50 kcal per lb) of body weight |
| 1–3 years | 100 kcal per kg (45 kcal per lb) of body weight |
| Over 3 years | 75–90 kcal per kg (35–40 kcal per lb) of body weight |

| | Girls | Boys |
|---|---|---|
| 13–15 years | 2600 kcal | 3200 kcal |
| 16–20 years | 2400 kcal | 3000 kcal |

### Man: Weight 63–70 kg

| | |
|---|---|
| Engaged in sedentary work | 2400 kcal |
| Engaged in active work | 3000 kcal |
| Engaged in heavy work | 4500 kcal |

### Woman: Weight 50–58 kg

| | |
|---|---|
| Engaged in sedentary work | 2000 kcal |
| Engaged in active work | 2400 kcal |
| Engaged in heavy work | 3000 kcal |
| During pregnancy | 2400 kcal |
| Breast-feeding a baby | 3000 kcal |

*Food*

An ideal diet of appropriate energy value should keep a person at the ideal weight for one of his age, height and build. The average or desirable weights of adults are recorded in this table:

**Average or Desirable Weights for Adults aged 30**

| Women<br>Height | | Small build | Medium build | Large build |
|---|---|---|---|---|
| 5′ 0″ | 1·52 m | 49·9 kg | 52·6 kg | 55·35 kg |
| 5′ 1″ | 1·55 m | 50·80 kg | 53·5 kg | 56·25 kg |
| 5′ 2″ | 1·57 m | 51·7 kg | 54·4 kg | 57·15 kg |
| 5′ 3″ | 1·60 m | 53·05 kg | 55·75 kg | 58·5 kg |
| 5′ 4″ | 1·63 m | 54·4 kg | 58·05 kg | 59·4 kg |
| 5′ 5″ | 1·65 m | 56·25 kg | 59·85 kg | 60·75 kg |
| 5′ 6″ | 1·68 m | 57·15 kg | 61·65 kg | 62·6 kg |
| 5′ 7″ | 1·70 m | 58·95 kg | 63·50 kg | 64·4 kg |
| 5′ 8″ | 1·73 m | 60·75 kg | 64·4 kg | 66·2 kg |
| 5′ 9″ | 1·75 m | 62·6 kg | 66·2 kg | 68·0 kg |
| 5′ 10″ | 1·78 m | 64·4 kg | 68·0 kg | 70·75 kg |

Plus or minus 1·35 kg for small build, 1·8 kg for medium build, and 2·25 kg for large build.

| Men<br>Height | | Small build | Medium build | Large build |
|---|---|---|---|---|
| 5′ 5″ | 1·65 m | 59·85 kg | 63·50 kg | 66·2 kg |
| 5′ 6″ | 1·68 m | 60·75 kg | 64·4 kg | 68·0 kg |
| 5′ 7″ | 1·70 m | 61·65 kg | 65·75 kg | 69·85 kg |
| 5′ 8″ | 1·73 m | 64·4 kg | 68·0 kg | 72·55 kg |
| 5′ 9″ | 1·75 m | 66·2 kg | 69·85 kg | 74·35 kg |
| 5′ 10″ | 1·78 m | 68·0 kg | 72·1 kg | 77·55 kg |
| 5′ 11″ | 1·80 m | 69·85 kg | 73·45 kg | 79·35 kg |
| 6′ 0″ | 1·83 m | 71·65 kg | 76·2 kg | 81·65 kg |
| 6′ 1″ | 1·85 m | 75·3 kg | 78·0 kg | 84·35 kg |
| 6′ 2″ | 1·88 m | 77·1 kg | 79·8 kg | 88·0 kg |

Plus or minus 1·8 kg for small build, 2·25 kg for medium build, and 2·7 kg for large build.

**Nutrition**

Nutrition is the nourishment of the tissues of the body. Among the factors that influence nutrition are:

1. The kinds of food eaten and its energy value.

2. The physical type of the person, who may naturally be slender, obese or muscular.

3. Physical illnesses, especially chronic infections of any kind.

4. Personal habits and physical activities in work or play.

5. Anxiety or other mental disturbance.

Most people in this country are now taller and better nourished than their ancestors, because they have better and more food, have better conditions to live and work in, have better health, and are freer from major infections.

**Malnutrition.** Some people are too thin. Their weight is below the normal weight for one of their age, sex and build, they are pale, they tire easily, their posture is poor, and they are liable to pick up infections more often than people of normal weight. Malnutrition may be due to poverty, ignorance, chronic ill health (such as may be caused by tuberculosis), or bad habits such as too little sleep, many late nights and smoking. Children may be thin because they have too little to eat, because they do not get enough protein in their diet to maintain normal development, because they are anxious or in other ways emotionally disturbed, or because they stay up too late at night or have too many out-of-school activities.

The treatment of malnutrition is by:

(a) Removal of the cause.

(b) Additions to the diet, especially of milk, butter, margarine, sugar, bread or chocolate as sources of energy; milk, meat, fish, liver and egg as sources of protein (50 per cent of an egg is composed of fat); increased vitamin intake, especially of fresh fruit and vegetables for ascorbic acid, halibut liver oil for vitamins A and D, and preparations of the vitamin B complex.

(c) Adequate sleep by night, and relaxation and rest periods by day.

(d) Moderate exercise as a stimulant to the tissues and to promote a healthy appetite, the exercise never being taken to the point of fatigue.

**Obesity.** Fat people often have a gross appetite, underdeveloped muscles and a bad posture, and are liable to develop diabetes, disease of the heart, and disease of the kidney. A person can be considered to be too fat when he is 20 per cent or more above the average weight for his height. It is better for people over the age of forty to be either of normal weight or slightly underweight, as the fatter middle-aged people are, the more likely are they to develop the diseases of obesity and the sooner will they die; and a person should aim at keeping his weight the same as it should be at the age of thirty or a little below it.

Obesity may be due to too rich a diet, to worry, which tends to make a person eat too much, to more sitting about and less exercise, or to a middle-aged decrease in thyroid activity and a consequently lower rate of metabolism in the tissues.

The treatment of obesity is by:

(a) A general reduction of the amount of food eaten, especially those of high energy value such as fat meat, rich cakes, fried potatoes and chocolate.

(b) A reduction in the amount of alcohol taken.

(c) Avoidance of worry as far as possible.

(d) Daily exercise in moderation.

**The Preparation and Cooking of Food.** Food should be fresh and uncontaminated. Where possible it should be kept in a refrigerator or cool larder and always protected from flies. It is very important that anyone handling food should keep their hands clean and their nails short; hands should always be washed after going to the lavatory and immediately before handling food.

All cooking vessels, crockery and cutlery should be kept clean. Detergents have now replaced soap as a cleansing agent in the kitchen. Crockery washed with a detergent should be swilled under a hot tap and stood to dry; it should not be dried on a teacloth, which may quickly become dirty or infected. Very small amounts of detergent powder are usually adequate. People whose hands are liable to develop a dermatitis on contact with a detergent should apply a wet barrier cream before washing up.

In houses cooking is usually done on an electric or gas stove. The larger kitchens of hospitals, hotels and canteens require more elaborate equipment of various kinds. In them steam is usually the main source of heating, being used for boiling vegetables, for preparing soups and sauces, and for heating the ovens in which puddings are cooked. Coke may be used for the baking ovens, where it gives a steady and constant temperature at an economical cost; gas stoves may be used for frying, boiling and grilling; fish and chip ranges may be heated by gas, coke or electric immersion-heaters; and in ultra-modern kitchens grilling may be done by infra-red rays.

Large kitchens should have adequate lavatory accommodation for the staff of each sex; a hand-basin and an electric hand-drier should be provided in each lavatory and the kitchen staff instructed and induced to use them on each visit. If an electrical hand-drier is not available, paper towels or continuous roller-towels, each person getting a clean piece of towel, should be provided.

# Chapter Four

# MILK

Cow's milk is drunk by babies when maternal milk is not available, by young children, and in lesser amounts by older children and adults. The differences in the chemical composition of human and cow's milk can be seen in these figures:

|  | *Percentage Composition* | |
|---|---|---|
|  | *Human Milk* | *Cow's Milk* |
| Protein | 1·7 | 3·2 |
| Lactose | 7·5 | 4·8 |
| Milk Fat | 3·5 | 3·7 |
| Mineral Salts | 0·2 | 0·7 |
| Water | 87·1 | 87·6 |

The composition of cow's milk varies with the breed of cow, its age, the season of the year and other factors; but where milk is supplied in bulk from many herds the average composition does not vary very much.

The milk of an animal is the one best suited to the rate of growth of its young and their digestive capabilities. A calf grows much more quickly than a baby, and cow's milk contains about twice as much protein and four times as much calcium as human milk. The curds formed by human milk in a baby's stomach are much softer and finer than those formed by cow's milk.

To maintain the quality of cow's milk, various regulations have been made. By law all milk sold must contain at least 3 per cent of fat and 8·5 per cent of solids other than fat. Channel Island Milk (from Jersey and Guernsey cows) and South Devon Milk (from South Devon cows) must contain at least 4 per cent of fat. Milk containing less than these proportions of fat or other solids is assumed to have been watered down or had some of its cream removed. Water, skimmed milk, preservatives or colouring matter must not be added to milk. Dairy farms and dairy farmers must be registered with the Ministry of Agriculture. Special regulations control 'attested herds' of tuberculin-tested cows. Milk from diseased cows must not be sold. Dairies and dairymen must be registered with the Local Authority, and dairy premises are subjected to inspection. The Community Physician can prohibit the sale of milk from premises where people suffering from infectious diseases live or work. Types of milk are designated by name, and the production of them and their subsequent treatment must conform to certain standards.

### Diseases spread by Milk

Breast-fed babies have the great advantage of being fed on fresh, sterile milk, given directly to them on demand from the producer. Cow's milk has two very serious disadvantages: micro-organisms can grow easily in it, and in its passage from producer (the cow) to consumer (a human being) it can easily become contaminated.

Diseases that can be spread by milk are:

1. *From diseased cows:* Tuberculosis, Undulant fever
2. *By contamination after leaving the cow:* Typhoid fever, Para-typhoid fever, Septic sore throat, Scarlet fever, Diphtheria

*Tuberculosis* was formerly very common in cows, and where milk is transported in bulk a lot of milk can be infected by a few cows. Efforts to reduce and abolish tuberculosis in cows have been very successful.

To reduce the incidence of tuberculosis in cows the following methods are used:

1. The building-up of 'attested herds' of cows negative to the tuberculin test.

2. The eradication of the disease from particular areas with the hope of bringing all the cows in the country up to the standard of the attested herds.

3. The slaughter of infected cows and the control of the movements of cows into healthy areas.

Pasteurization and sterilization are the most effective ways of making sure that milk drunk is not infected with the tubercle bacillus.

*Undulant Fever* is due to the infection of cows with *Brucella abortus*. In them the disease is known as contagious abortion. The micro-organisms are killed by pasteurization or sterilization.

*Typhoid Fever, Paratyphoid Fever, Septic Sore Throat, Scarlet Fever and Diphtheria* can be caused by the infection of milk by a person suffering from one of these diseases or being a carrier of one of them. The micro-organisms that cause these diseases are destroyed by pasteurization and sterilization.

**The Farm.** The herd should be healthy. A good cow yields from two to three gallons a day. Cows are milked twice daily, in the early morning and in the afternoon; with a milking machine one man should be able to milk thirty cows. The cow-sheds should be clean, well lighted and airy. The walls and floors should be made of impervious material. The shed should be washed daily and, if it is not tiled, whitewashed every six months. The cows should not have to walk through manure on the way to be milked. Dung from the cow should drop into a gutter, from which it can be washed away. The udder, teats and flanks should be wiped with a damp cloth before milking. The milker should wear clean overalls and cap, and should wash his hands before beginning to milk. All milk pails and churns should be sterilized by steam. The milk should be cooled immediately. It is either sold in bulk to dairies in the towns or bottled for sale off the farm.

*Tuberculin-tested milk* is milk from special 'attested herds', registered with the Ministry of Agriculture. All cows in the herd must be negative to tuberculin, be inspected at intervals by a veterinary surgeon, and be kept apart from other cows.

*Attested Areas.* Thanks to the efforts of farmers, veterinary surgeons, and the Government veterinary services, the whole of England, Wales and Scotland is now an 'attested area', in which all cattle are tested for freedom from tuberculosis.

**Dairies.** Milk is taken in churns from the farms to the country depots of the dairy companies. There the quality of the milk is tested by smell, samples of doubtful milk are examined in the laboratory, and unsatisfactory milk is rejected. In addition, each farmer's milk is regularly examined for its fat content and content of solids other than fat. If the milk has to be taken to a central depot, it is cooled and put into 3,000-gallon transport tankers of stainless steel or glass-lined steel, insulated so effectively that the temperature of the milk in them does not rise more than one or two degrees during the journey.

At the central depot the milk is treated by heat to destroy organisms and make it keep longer. The two methods of heat treatment are pasteurization and sterilization.

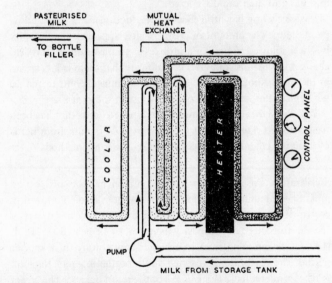

FIG. 1. *Milk pasteurization plant*

**Pasteurization.** Pasteurization (called after the French bacterio-logist, Pasteur) is the heating of milk to a definite temperature for a certain length of time, followed by cooling and automatic bottle-filling (see Fig. 1). In this way all harmful bacteria are destroyed and the number of milk-souring organisms reduced, the milk being rendered safe to drink and keeping longer than raw milk.

The High-Temperature-Short-Time (H-T-S-T) method is the one commonly used. In this method the milk is heated to 161° F

(72° C) for fifteen seconds and then immediately cooled to approximately 40° F (4·5° C). The cold pasteurized milk is at once fed automatically into milk bottles that have been washed and sterilized. The bottles are automatically capped with aluminium foil, which must overlap the pouring lip of the bottle.

The Holder Method is the older method of pasteurization, now replaced in many plants by the H-T-S-T method, which can pasteurize a much larger quantity of milk in a day. In the Holder Method the milk is kept at a temperature of 145° F (63° C) for thirty minutes and then rapidly cooled.

Pasteurization has little effect on the food-value of milk and its palatability. The amount of cream which appears after the milk has been allowed to stand is a little less, but this is due to physical changes in the milk and does not indicate that there is less cream in the milk. About 20 per cent of the vitamin C content and 10 per cent of the vitamin D content is lost in the process.

*T.T. Pasteurized Milk* is milk from attested herds that has been pasteurized. *Channel Island Pasteurized Milk* is milk from herds of Channel Island Cows pasteurized by the same methods.

**Sterilization.** Pasteurization is the common method of treating milk by heat, but some people prefer it sterilized. Sterilization destroys all micro-organisms in milk. Sterilized milk has to pass a special 'turbidity test', to pass which it must be heated to 212° F (100° C) for ten minutes or to a higher temperature for a shorter period. The sterilization is carried out in bottles in which the milk will keep indefinitely as long as the bottle is not opened. The cream becomes intimately mixed in the milk and does not settle out on top of the milk on standing. The high temperature to which the milk is heated produces a slightly cooked flavour and a slightly brown tint; its food value is only slightly reduced.

**Homogenized milk** is milk that has been subjected to a process that intimately mixes cream and milk, after which no cream settles out on standing. After homogenization the milk is pasteurized in one of the usual ways. Homogenized milk is often supplied to hospitals, hotels and catering establishments as no stirring is necessary to keep the cream evenly distributed.

## Precautions in the Home

1. Milk should not be left standing in bottles for long on a door-step because it goes stale and the vitamin C in it is quickly destroyed by exposure to sunlight.

2. Milk should be kept in the bottle until it is required. It should be kept in a refrigerator or cool larder. Milk jugs should be covered with muslin caps when they are not in a refrigerator.

3. A milk bottle should be rinsed out in cold water as soon as it has been emptied. This stops micro-organisms and moulds growing in it and flies from laying eggs in it; some flies lay eggs which adhere very firmly to the inside of the bottle and cannot be removed by ordinary washing methods.

4. The bottle should not be used for any other purpose and should be returned promptly to the milkman.

## Milk Products

*Dried Milk* is the white powder left when all the water in milk is driven out by heat. The powder contains all the foodstuffs of milk, and when the right amount of water is added to it milk is re-formed. There are two main methods of manufacture: (a) the Roller method, in which the milk is dried by being run over heated rollers; and (b) the Spray method, in which the milk is sprayed into hot air. Dried milk is commonly used as a baby food; it has the great advantages of being sterile and keeping for a long time. Some dried milks are prepared from milk from which the cream has been partly or wholly removed; the label on the tin describes the contents as being from full, $\frac{3}{4}$, $\frac{1}{2}$ or $\frac{1}{4}$ cream milk or from skimmed milk. Vitamin D is added to dried milk; the dose now recommended is 100 international units per dry ounce.

*Condensed Milk* is milk from which part of the water has been removed by heat. To re-form milk from it, water has to be added in certain amounts. There are two kinds of condensed milk: (a) sweetened condensed milk, to which sugar has been added; and (b) unsweetened 'evaporated' milk.

*Cream* is the part of the milk rich in fat. It can be separated from milk by skimming and other methods. Its bacterial content being high, it should be pasteurized.

*Skimmed Milk* is milk from which the cream has been removed.

# Chapter Five

# HOUSES

One of the ways of keeping healthy is to live in a good house. Bad houses and disease commonly go together: rates of sickness and death are much higher in slums than in good housing estates. This association may be partly due to conditions other than housing, such as the poverty and low intelligence of many of the inhabitants of slums and bad houses. Into such a bad house sunlight and air may not easily enter; the house may be dirty, neglected and in bad repair; its drains may be defective; it may lack bath and lavatory, space to hang clothes up to dry, and a garden for children to play in.

Although many slums have been pulled down and replaced by modern housing estates, there are still many old houses that do not come up to the standards of good modern housing.

To be satisfactory a house should be dry, warm and in a state of good repair. It should have:

(a) drinking water available inside the house and adequate facilities for heating water;

(b) satisfactory places for storing, preparing and cooking food;

(c) sinks, a bath and a lavatory;

(d) an adequate drainage system;

(e) adequate lighting, natural and artificial;

(f) adequate ventilation and facilities for heating each room;

(g) a place to store fuel;

(h) access to outbuildings, and a back door to the street as well as a front door.

One of the major difficulties in designing and equipping a house in this country is the provision of adequate warmth in the winter. Ideally all the rooms in the house would be so warm that any member of the family could be able to do what he wants to without interfering with other members of the family. Such an ideal would entail some form of central heating; but the expense of installing the equipment and of maintaining it in fuel makes central heating expensive for the ordinary household, many of whom can afford to keep only one room really warm during the winter.

**Sites.** In the selection of a site for a house, a housing estate, a hospital or other building, several factors have to be considered, such as the kinds of land available, their cost, and the convenience of the site for the purposes of the building and for the people who are going to live or work in it.

A site for a house or hospital should be open in aspect, dry, sunny, freely exposed to air, and with a slight gradient in at least one direction, so that natural currents will cause air to circulate around and so that drainage is easy to provide.

A very important factor in building is the nature of the subsoil, the ground immediately beneath the top layer of soil. The best sites are those with a dry and porous subsoil, through which rain-water can pass freely. Subsoils of gravel, sandstone, chalk, rock and slate are usually dry and suitable for building on. Unsuitable sites for building on are: wet clay; low-lying land likely to become water-logged; sand lying above an impervious layer and therefore likely to be wet; land that has been built up by rubbish-tipping; and alluvial subsoil, which is ground washed down by a river or stream.

### Building Construction

Houses in this country are usually made of brick, stone or wood: and although traditional designs and methods of construction have recently been challenged by new ideas and materials, the basic principles of building remain the same.

The *Foundations* are very important. They must be strong and wide enough to take the weight of the building and all its contents without causing any sinking of the subsoil, an occurrence that would make the house settle unevenly. The foundations of an ordinary house are made of concrete at least 9 inches deep and wider by at least 6 inches on each side than the bricks laid upon it.

Concrete is a mixture of cement with small pieces of brick and stone, sand and water, hardening to a very firm solid and

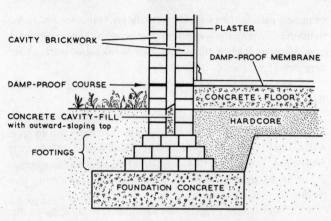

FIG. 2. *Diagram showing foundations and wall construction of a house*

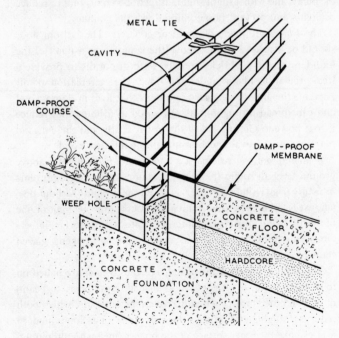

FIG. 3. *Diagram showing cavity wall construction*

commonly used for foundations, walls, floors, staircases and roofs. 'Reinforced concrete' is concrete strengthened by having steel rods set in it; it is used where the concrete has to take strains other than mere weight.

The spaces between the foundations of a building are usually filled by concrete or asphalt.

The *Walls* of a house or small building are usually made of brick. The best are 'cavity walls', which are made of an inner and an outer wall of brick with an air-space between them (see Fig. 3). A cavity wall helps to keep a house dry, warm in winter, and cool in summer.

The cavity may be filled with materials with insulating properties.

A *Chimney* from a fireplace should be at least 9 inches in diameter, plastered inside to present a smooth surface to the outflow of smoke, and with a slight shift in direction at one point to reduce draughts and prevent rain coming down the chimney.

The *Floors* are made of wood or concrete. The bottom floor should be at least 3 inches above the concrete or asphalt of the foundation; and air-bricks must be set in the walls to provide a free circulation of air under the floor. Free circulation of air prevents the growth of *dry rot*, a fungus that lives in damp wood and can spread throughout all the wood in a house and reduce it to a powder. Getting rid of dry rot is costly and difficult and may involve removal and burning all the infected wood.

A *damp-proof course* must be built in the walls a little above ground level all round the house. A damp-proof course prevents moisture from rising up in the wall from the ground; without one, a house is liable to become damp. The course must be built of one of the following impervious materials: slates set in mortar; impervious blue bricks set in mortar; sheet lead set in cement; glazed slabs or bricks; bituminous felt.

The *Roof* is usually made of slates or tiles, which are nailed on to wooden battens (strips of wood fastened from beam to beam) or laid on boards with a felt undercovering, a measure which both reduces draughts and reduces the risk of freezing. Some modern houses have the inner surface of the boards lined with aluminium sheeting for the same purposes. The cistern and its connecting pipes are commonly put under the roof. If they are unprotected, the water in them is likely to freeze, particularly if the spaces between the beams of the top ceiling of the house have been filled with fibre-glass or some other heat-impervious substance in order to prevent the heat in the house being lost through the roof. If the cistern and pipes are under the roof, they should be 'lagged' with asbestos or felt to prevent the water freezing in them during frosts.

*Large buildings*, such as hospitals, factories and blocks of flats and offices, are usually built as steel-framed buildings. The steel frame makes a skeleton of vertical and horizontal girders, through which the weight of the building is transmitted to the foundations. In buildings thus constructed no weight is transmitted through the walls, which can in consequence be thin and light.

**Keeping Out the Damp.** Keeping the damp out of a house is very important. A damp house is a cold house, difficult to heat and depressing to anyone living in it; damp damages the structure of the house and any furniture or textiles it contains. The three principal causes of damp in a house are building damp, condensation and rain-water.

*Building Damp* occurs in new houses and is due to the water in the plaster of the walls coming through into the rooms. With natural ventilation it will disappear in a few months; central heating hastens its departure. Ideally a house should not be lived in until it has 'dried out', but because of the housing shortage people usually move into a house as soon as the building is finished.

*Condensation* is due to water vapour forming drops of water on cold windows and walls. It can be prevented by efficient ventilation.

*Rain-water* can get into a house through the roof, through the walls, and from the ground. Roof damp is usually due to defective slates, to too narrow eaves (the projecting edges of the roof), to defective gutters, or to bad joins where the slates meet the chimneys. Cavity walls prevent damp getting in through the walls. Where a house has not got cavity walls, the outside can be coated with mortar, which can be pebble-dashed, or covered with slates or tiles. Rain-water pipes and guttering should be kept in good repair. To prevent damp rising through the walls from the ground, an adequate damp-proof course should be inserted in the walls when the house is being built.

**Prevention of Accidents.** When houses are built or repaired attention must be paid to the avoidance of accidents by people who have to live in them, particularly old people. The house, especially the stairs, should be well lit, and light switches should be placed in easily accessible positions; there should be a light switch by each bedside so that a person, getting out of bed, does not have to go across the room in the dark. Chimneys should not be obstructed, and fires should be fitted by experts, so that poisonous products do not enter the room. In the kitchen the cooker should be next to the sink and not on the opposite side, so that a person does not have to carry pans of hot liquids across the room. Baths should have rails at the sides so that old people can pull themselves up, or a shallow bath should be put in from which the feeble can easily get out. The stairs should be kept in good condition and the hand-rail must be firm; a little knob may be inserted into the hand-rail in such a position that a person going downstairs knows by touching the knob that he has actually reached the bottom. Windows through which children might fall should be guarded.

# Chapter Six

# AIR AND VENTILATION

Air is a mixture of gases in the following approximate proportions:

| | |
|---|---|
| Oxygen | 21 per cent |
| Carbon dioxide | 0·04 per cent |
| Nitrogen | 78 per cent |
| Argon and other gases | 1 per cent |

This is the air we breathe in—inspired air. Expired air, the air we breathe out, has had some oxygen removed and some carbon dioxide added, with the result that these two gases occur in it in different proportions:

| | |
|---|---|
| Oxygen | 16 per cent |
| Carbon dioxide | 4 per cent |

In addition to these gases air contains a small amount of water vapour, the amount of which varies from day to day and place to place. The pressure of the atmosphere at sea-level is 14·7 lb. per square inch (or one atmosphere), but we are not aware of this pressure nor crushed by it because it is transmitted equally in all directions.

The impurities that can occur in air are:

*Dust*, organic or inorganic, from fires, roads, factories, building demolition and decaying vegetable matter.

*Smoke*, from fires.

*Pollen*, from plants and grasses.

*Bacteria*, dead and alive.

*Sulphur dioxide* and *sulphuric acid*, from factories.

*Carbon monoxide*, from fires and car exhausts.

These impurities are removed from the air by the action of the sun, the wind and the rain.

**Air Pollution.** Fresh air, light and sunshine are essential for health and normal growth; many pathogenic organisms can be killed by light and air, and sunshine can prevent and cure rickets. Everybody knows how much better they feel on a bright sunny day compared to a dull overcast one. Air pollution can be a very serious threat to health. The chief causes of pollution are smoke from domestic, uses and industry, carbon monoxide from car exhausts, and various chemicals from factories.

*Smoke* is a mixture of carbon, grit, dust, sulphur dioxide and tar in proportions that vary with the nature of the coal or fuel burnt and the method by which it is burnt. The carbon in smoke is produced by imperfect combustion. In perfect combustion each atom of carbon combines with two atoms of oxygen to form carbon dioxide, which is invisible; in imperfect combustion unburnt particles of carbon are discharged into the air. The amount of grit and dust in smoke is usually much greater than the amount of carbon in it. Sulphur dioxide, a gaseous product of the combustion of solid, liquid and gaseous fuels, combines with moisture in the atmosphere to form weak sulphuric acid and is the 'killer' substance in 'smog'. Smoke reduces the amount of sunshine that reaches the earth, causes a deposit of carbon in the lungs and thoracic lymph glands, retards the growth of vegetables, and seriously damages the stonework of buildings. People living in a smoke-polluted atmosphere are liable to develop rhinitis, sinusitis and chronic bronchitis—the 'English disease' of today. Smoke pollution appears in its most dangerous form as 'smog', that dense mixture of smoke and fog that is liable to occur in cities under certain climatic conditions. Smog can have very harmful effects upon the respiratory systems of the very young, the old, and chronic respiratory or cardiac invalids. In three December weeks of 'smog' in London in 1952 about 4,000 people are believed to have died of its effects. A similar but shorter and less severe 'smog' in London produced over 1,000 deaths, and similar catastrophes have been reported in other parts of the world.

It is generally assumed that factory chimneys are the chief source of smoke, but this is no longer true. It has been estimated that in Britain in 1973 the total emitted from domestic sources was 0·44 million metric tonnes and from industrial sources 0·08 million metric tonnes. The reduction of smoke from all sources is therefore a major hygienic measure intended to reduce the incidence and severity of many chest diseases.

*The Clean Air Act, 1956*, was introduced as a measure to reduce the smoke nuisance to a minimum. One of its sections gives a Local Authority the power to establish 'smokeless areas' in which householders must burn smokeless fuels. Another prohibits the emission of 'dark smoke' from the chimneys of houses, factories, shops and offices, and from the funnels of ships and railway locomotives. 'Dark smoke' is defined as smoke as dark as or darker than Shade 2 on the Ringelmann Chart. The Ringelmann Chart, designed many years ago by a French professor, is a card graduated from 0 (white, no smoke) to 1 (light grey), 2 (darker grey), 3 (very dark grey), 4 (black) and 5 (dense black), and in use is held fifty feet from the observer and in line with the chimney being tested. Although house chimneys are included in the ban, they rarely produce smoke as dark as Shade 2.

Although the ordinary old-fashioned open coal fire may not produce dark smoke it can pollute the air by discharging unburnt particles of carbon into it. In modern grates the back is designed to direct the smoke over the flames in which much of it is consumed. The slow-combustion stove and domestic boiler produces less smoke because the amount of air entering them can be controlled and because they burn smokeless fuels such as coke and anthracite.

In the usual steam-boiler furnaces used in factories and other large buildings the amount of smoke discharged can be reduced by regulation of the air entry, mechanical stoking, forced draughts to improve combustion, and devices to remove dust, grit and unburnt carbon before the smoke is discharged into the air.

### Ventilation

Ventilation is the free passage of air. Air is kept moving by natural influences—the sun, the wind and the rain. By warming land and sea the sun produces air currents and winds, which by their movements keep constant the composition of the air; the rain washes to the ground the carbon and other impurities of the air.

The ventilation of a house is the removal of impure air and its replacement by pure air. This requires the replacement of all the air in a room at least twice an hour, and for the comfort of its inhabitants and the slow burning of its fires the air has to be changed without a draught being produced. Moreover the ventilation of a house cannot be considered apart from its heating, with which ventilation is closely allied.

Rooms are normally ventilated by their windows, doors and chimneys (see Fig. 4). This natural ventilation is controlled by

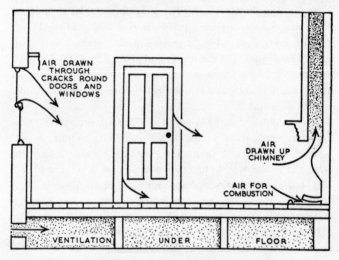

FIG. 4. *Diagram showing ventilation in a room*

differences between the temperature inside and outside the house. Air usually enters a room by the windows or by cracks around the windows and door and goes out up the chimney. When a fire is out, the wind blowing across the top of the chimney extracts the air in the chimney, and the chimney draws air from the room; when the fire is lit the effects are increased by warm air rising up the chimney.

An electric fan, built into a window or an outside wall, may be used for both extracting air from a room and discharging it into the atmosphere and bringing in fresh air from outside (see Fig. 5).

Such a fan is especially useful in a kitchen, a scullery and a bath-room. In large buildings an electric fan may be placed in an air-trunk used to conduct air to many rooms.

The cubic capacity of a room is obtained by multiplying the length by the breadth and the height up to a maximum of 12 feet, the height above 12 feet not being taken into consideration for ven-tilation estimates. Certain minimum cubic capacities for rooms,

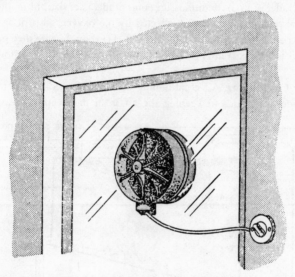

FIG. 5. *Electric fan in a window*

wards, factories, lodging houses, etc., are approved; every patient in a general hospital, for example, should have at least 1,200 cubic feet of space and every patient in a maternity hospital 2,000 cubic feet; but arrangements based on these figures have the weakness of not taking into consideration the type and efficiency of the ven-tilation provided.

**Effects of Inefficient Ventilation.** Comfort in a room depends mainly upon the area of wall space available to receive the heat radiated off the bodies of the people within it. It is this heat that may make the atmosphere of a room uncomfortable. Moreover moisture and smells from bodies and clothing become more noticeable, especially by people coming into the room. In hot rooms people perspire more and their clothes become moist. In a badly ventilated room the body becomes hot and sweaty, the temperature of the room rises, people are likely to become tired, to yawn, to sleep or even to faint. Living for long periods in ill-ventilated rooms leads to debility, loss of appetite and loss of energy.

Under normal conditions, in rooms of adequate size, the amount of oxygen in the air is not affected by the oxygen absorption of the people in it, and the slight amount of carbon dioxide they produce is not of any importance and does not produce any symptoms.

**Air Conditioning.** Air conditioning is the term used to describe modern methods of keeping the air fresh in cinemas, theatres

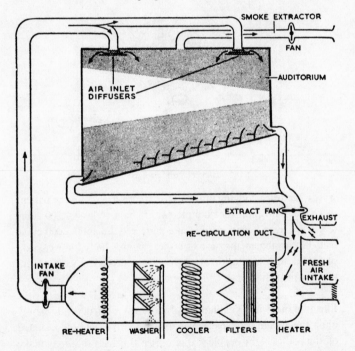

FIG. 6. *Air-conditioning plant in a cinema*

hospitals, hotels and other large buildings. An air-conditioning plant keeps the air in constant circulation by means of electric pumps, filters off dust, removes gases, adds water vapour, and warms or cools it to the required temperature (see Fig. 6).

The plant consists of (a) an entrance for fresh air from the atmosphere, (b) a filter to remove gross particles, (c) a heater to heat the air so that it will pick up moisture in the next stage, (d) a series of water sprays to add water vapour, (e) eliminator plates to remove dirt and particles of water, and (f) further heaters to bring the air to the appropriate temperature. After this treatment the air is pumped through several inlets into the hall or rooms where it is required. From the hall the stale air is sucked out by other pumps and discharged into the atmosphere or into the conditioning plant for treatment and further circulation.

# Chapter Seven

# HEATING AND LIGHTING

Heating and ventilation make buildings fit for people to live and work in and for materials to be stored. The technical name for the artificial heating of buildings is 'space-heating'. Methods of space-heating depend upon the climate, the mode of life of people, the kinds of fuel available and their costs, the methods of building, and the amount of scientific knowledge on the subject.

Heat is conveyed from one thing or place to another in three ways: radiation, convection and conduction. *Radiation* is the transfer of heat without material contact between the body that loses heat and the one that gains heat, e.g. from an open coal fire. *Convection* is the transfer of heat by actual movement of the heated material, e.g. the movement of water in a domestic system or the rising of hot air from the top of a stove. Most methods of heating use both radiation and convection. The third method, *conduction*, which is the transfer of heat from one thing to another without the parts moving, e.g. the transfer of heat from a gas-ring to a saucepan, is not used in space-heating.

The main sources of heat are coal, coke, electricity, gas and oil. They are used to produce hot air, hot water or steam.

The two main types of heating systems are:

1. *Direct Heating*. Heat is generated in the room where it is required.

2. *Indirect Heating*. The fuel is burned in one place and the heat conducted from it to other rooms or houses. It is called *central heating* when it is applied to one house, and *district heating* when it is used for several houses or buildings.

## Direct Heating

The *open coal fire* is a cheerful and dirty luxury. It is inefficient, for it requires much attention and throws out into the room only about 25 per cent of the heat-energy in the coal, and it is dirty because it produces smoke. Its efficiency has been improved and its production of smoke diminished by improvements in the shape of the fire-clay back, which by throwing the escaping gases and smoke forwards radiates heat into the room and ensures that many of the carbon particles in the smoke are consumed. Because coal fires need a lot of air they produce draughts.

*Slow combustion stoves* are designed to burn coal or coke. The air intake into them is regulated by a damper at the bottom, which enables the heat produced by this stove to be much more under control than that from an open fire. The production of smoke can be slight and the fire can burn for many hours without attention. Such stoves are about 70 per cent efficient. The heat from them is mainly by the convection of hot air and partly, when the doors of the stove are open, by radiation (see Fig. 7).

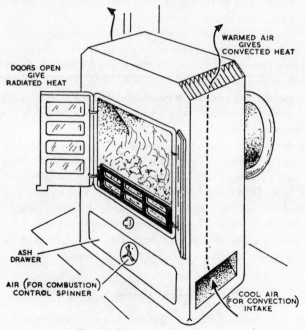

FIG. 7. *Slow combustion stove*

*Gas stoves* are made of elements called radiants, which are heated to a white heat by a row of bunsen burners below them. They are about 50 per cent efficient. *Convector gas fires* are much more efficient, for in addition to heating a room by radiation from elements, they draw air in at the base, heat it and discharge it into the room, warming it by convection; the gases from the radiants are discharged into the chimney (see Fig. 8).

For open fires, stoves and gas fires a chimney is essential for the removal of the products of combustion. The chimney should be at least 12 feet high and 9 inches in its internal diameter. It should come out as near the ridge of the roof as possible in order to prevent down draughts (currents of air passing down the chimney into the room). Soot inside a chimney may catch fire; but chimneys are so made, of brick or stone, that whatever the temperature (even when it is on fire) the outside of the chimney never becomes hot enough to set the house on fire. To prevent fires, the chimney should be swept at least once a year.

*Electric fires* produce heat by the passage of an electric current through wires of metal resistant to electricity. The whole of the energy is liberated for use and the efficiency is 100 per cent. Electric fires have the advantages of being clean, requiring little attention, heating up rapidly, requiring no chimney and being portable. The best kinds have reflectors with a highly polished surface reflecting all the heat produced.

Other methods of electrical heating are: radiators enclosing oil and heated by electrical elements; tubular and panel heaters fixed to walls or ceilings; tubes laid in the concrete of the foundations of a house; and electrically heated underlays for carpets.

*Oil stoves* are used where other methods of heating cannot be employed or as an accessory to other heating. They are often used to provide a low 'background' heat. They should be used only where there is adequate ventilation through a window or chimney.

### Indirect Heating

The usual methods of central and district heating employ hot air, steam or hot water. The fuel may be coke, gas, oil, or crude tar.

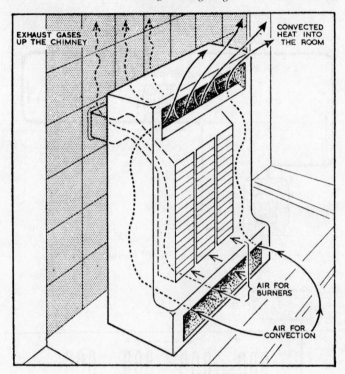

FIG. 8. *Convector gas fire*

*Hot Air.* From a thermostatically-controlled stove on the ground floor or in a basement, hot air is directed through flues to the rooms to be warmed.

*Steam.* Steam is often used for factories, hospitals and other large buildings. It may be used with or without radiators. The steam may be under low pressure or, where heat has to be transmitted long distances, under high pressure. Steam-heating has the disadvantages of making pipes and radiators very hot and of not being easily adjusted to daily variation in temperature.

*Hot Water.* Hot water is a common method of heating houses. A boiler in the basement or on the ground floor heats the water in a jacket around it, and as the water becomes hot it rises through pipes to the top of the house. As it loses its heat and is replaced

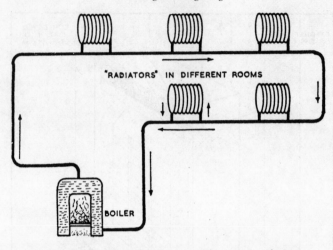

FIG. 9. *Diagram showing central heating in a house*

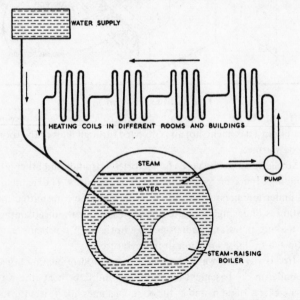

FIG. 10. *High pressure hot-water system*

by hotter water from the boiler, it passes downwards by gravity, going through radiators which it heats. It is then returned to the boiler to be reheated and resume the circuit (see Fig. 9).

Radiators are frequently placed under windows to heat the air as it enters the room. They are made of a series of fluted tubes through which the water passes. The word 'radiator' is a misnomer, as most of the heat is given off by convection.

*High-pressure Hot-Water Systems.* These are used for heating large buildings, the hot water being heated under pressure in a steam-raising boiler and pumped through the heating system (see Fig. 10).

**Measurement of Heat.** A British Thermal Unit (B.T.U.) can be defined as the amount of heat required to raise the temperature of 1 lb of water by $1°$ F. It is equal to $1·055$ kilojoules (kJ). A *therm* is 100,000 B.T.U.s, i.e. $105·5$ megajoules (MJ). A *unit* of electricity is 1 kilowatt hour (kW h) = $3·6$ megajoules (MK) or 3,412 B.T.U.s.

The temperature of a ward should be $16-18°$ C ($60-64°$ F). The temperature of an operating theatre should be between 21 and $27°$C ($70-80°$ F). The temperature of a sitting-room should be about $16°$ C ($60°$ F).

**Installing a Heating System.** The choice of a heating system is best left to a heating engineer. Among the factors he will consider are:

The type of building to be heated and its purpose
The temperature required
The types of fuel available
Combinations of direct and indirect heating
The cost of installation
The costs of maintenance, labour and repairs

The approximate efficiency of the various types of heating are:

| | |
|---|---|
| open coal fire | 25 per cent |
| gas fire | 50-65 per cent |
| anthracite stove | 70 per cent |
| electric fire | 100 per cent |
| coke central heating | 60 per cent |
| gas central heating | 70 per cent |
| oil central heating | 85 per cent |

**Hot Water.** The method used to produce heat for the house may also be used to produce hot water for washing and bathing and heat for cooking. Multi-purpose units exist in various forms, especially in small houses, where one fire may be used to heat the living-room, to do the cooking and to provide hot water. Other combinations provide hot water for both washing and central heating.

Other methods of heating water are:

1. An *Electric Immersion Heater.* A rod made of a resistant metal, surrounded by insulating material and encased in a metal tube, the whole being inserted in the hot-water tank. The heater is thermostatically controlled so that it maintains the water at a determined temperature.

2. A *Large-Scale Thermal Unit.* A central storage vessel is heated by electricity at night (when electricity costs less) and the hot water stored for use by day. The central heating systems of large buildings such as hospitals and blocks of flats may be supplied in the same way.

## Lighting

Lighting may be natural or artificial. Natural light comes from the sun; artificial light is almost everywhere in this country provided by electricity.

Lighting should be:

(a) adequate for the work done by it;

(b) uniform and constant;

(c) so arranged that shadows are not cast on the work done;

(d) so arranged that there is no 'glare', i.e. that the source of the light does not shine directly into the eyes nor is reflected into them off a shiny surface.

Illumination is measured in so many 'lumens' per unit area, usually a square foot or square metre. The following are some of the recommended amounts of light for various kinds of work:

|  | $1m/ft^2$ | $1m/m^2$ |
|---|---|---|
| Reading and writing | 7–30 | 75–320 |
| Domestic work | 7 | 75 |
| Sewing | 20 | 215 |

| | lm/ft² | lm/m² |
|---|---|---|
| Engineering drawing | 30 | 323 |
| Ward, general | 3 | 32 |
| Ward, bed | 15 | 161 |
| Operating theatre | 30 | 323 |
| Operating table | 300 | 3,230 |

**Natural Lighting.** The amount of natural light in a room depends upon the amount of sunlight outside and the shape, size and position of the windows. For the same window-area, windows give better light if they are high rather than low and wide; and the amount of light falling on to horizontal surfaces such as tables and beds comes mainly through the upper parts of the windows. Where as much natural light as possible is required, such as in a ward or working room, windows should reach to the top of the walls.

Pale wall-papers and paints on internal walls improve natural lighting by reflecting and diffusing light and making brighter the walls in which the windows are set.

**Artificial Lighting.** Artificial lighting should be planned to suit the main purposes of a room, its shape, size and contents. In general the main work done should be as brightly illuminated as the general field of vision. Deep shadows should be avoided, but some shadow is helpful in producing contrast.

The electric tungsten bulb is the commonest source of light used. It consists of a very fine tungsten wire, coiled into a small spiral and connected with wires in the neck of the bulb. The lamp is filled with an inert gas—nitrogen or argon—in which a higher temperature can be achieved than the vacuum formerly used. Light is produced by the passage of the electric current through the tungsten wire.

Light from the bulb may be *direct*—the rays of light falling directly upon the work (with a shade where necessary to prevent them from shining directly into the eyes); *indirect*—the light being reflected from ceiling or wall by an opaque bowl below the bulb; or *semi-direct*—part of the light coming through a semi-opaque bowl and part reflected from ceiling and wall, a method that gives, when an electric bulb is used, the minimum of glare and shadow.

*Fluorescent lighting* is replacing the tungsten bulb in public places. A fluorescent lamp has a long glass tube, coated inside with a mixture of chemical substances called phosphors and filled with argon and a little mercury. An electrical discharge through the lamp produces ultra-violet light, and this ultra-violet light causes the phosphors to produce a brilliant light, which is free from glare and casts little shadow. The colour of the light depends upon the composition of the phosphors; daylight and other 'white' lights can be produced where required.

Electricity as a source of light has the advantages of being clean and free from smell and using no oxygen.

**Lighting a Ward.** In a hospital ward the lighting should provide:

(a) general lighting without glare; this is best done by fluorescent lighting;

(b) individual lighting for each bed, so that patients can read or sew; this is best done by semi-opaque wall-lights above the beds;

(c) a dim, diffused light at night so that the nurse may see her patients without their being kept awake by too bright a light.

At convenient intervals points should be fitted to which special lamps or other pieces of electrical equipment can be fitted.

# Chapter Eight

# WATER SUPPLIES

Water is a chemical substance whose molecules are composed of two parts of hydrogen and one part of oxygen; its chemical formula is $H_2O$. It can exist in three forms—as a liquid (water), as a solid (ice) and as a gas (steam). At ordinary atmospheric pressure at sea-level water freezes and becomes ice when its temperature falls to $32°$ F ($0°$ C). As it freezes it expands to about one-tenth more than its original volume; this expansion will burst a pipe, from which the water will escape when the ice melts. At ordinary atmospheric pressure water boils and turns to steam when its temperature rises to $212°$ F ($100°$ C). One of the characteristic properties of water is its ability to dissolve other substances. As a result of this natural water is never chemically pure, for rain will both absorb impurities in the atmosphere as it falls and disssolve chemical substances as it passes through the ground.

Rain, hail and snow are the sources of all the water used. When rain falls on the earth, one of three things happens to it:

(a) it may evaporate and return to the atmosphere;

(b) it may run off the surface of the ground and form streams, rivers and lakes;

(c) it may sink down through the soil until it reaches an impervious layer through which it cannot pass, and from which it runs into springs, deep wells, and the bed of rivers and lakes.

Snow provides a rich supply of water to the earth, for the deeper layers of it are melted by the warmth of the earth, and the water thus produced sinks into the ground.

Water is necessary to man for many purposes:

*For Domestic Use:* drinking, washing, cooking, house-cleaning, laundry, lavatories, gardening.

*For Trades:* necessary for many trades.

*For Municipal Use:* washing streets, washing sewers, public lavatories, municipal baths and swimming baths, public gardens and parks, fire services.

The amount of water consumed in towns is increasing. About 100 gallons of water per person per day are provided in English and Welsh towns for all purposes—domestic, trade and municipal. In many American towns the average figure is over 100 gallons. A little over half the total amount is used for domestic purposes. total amount is used for domestic purposes.

**Good Water.** It is essential that people should be provided with water that is adequate in amount, constant in its supply, pure and wholesome.

Good drinking water should:

1. Have no taste, smell or colour.
2. Be sparkling.
3. Contain no nitrogenous organic matter.
4. Not be infected with harmful micro-organisms.
5. Not contain poisonous metals.

**Fluoridation.** This is the term used to describe the addition of fluoride to water. The addition of fluoride in the form of sodium fluoride or sodium silicofluoride can do much to prevent dental caries. The concentration should not be more than one part per million, as stronger concentrations can produce a mottling of the enamel of the teeth.

**Hard and Soft Water.** As rain passes through the atmosphere it picks up ammonia, carbon dioxide and (in industrial areas) sulphuric acid. As it percolates through the ground it dissolves (because of the carbon dioxide in it) calcium carbonate in the form of soluble calcium bicarbonate. Calcium sulphate and magnesium sulphate and also calcium chloride and magnesium chloride may also be dissolved out of the ground. The absorption of calcium will be greatest when the water passes through chalky soil.

Water is said to be 'hard' when it contains an excess of calcium and magnesium. The 'hardness' is measured in degrees, one degree being equal to 1 grain of calcium per gallon of water. A 'soft water' has a hardness of about 5 degrees, a 'hard water' may have a hardness of 20 degrees.

Hard water is a nuisance because it prevents soap from lathering (forming an insoluble curd on skin and basin), produces 'fur' in kettles and 'scale' in boilers, discharges the green out of vegetables, and toughens meat cooked in it.

Rain and upland waters are soft; river water varies from soft to hard; well water is hard.

'Temporary hardness' is due to calcium bicarbonate, and is called temporary because the hardness disappears when the water is boiled, carbon dioxide being driven off into the air and calcium carbonate being deposited as fur or scale.

'Permanent hardness' is due to dissolved sulphates and chlorides of calcium and magnesium and is not affected by boiling. It may be slightly reduced by the addition of washing soda (sodium carbonate) to the water. Hard water may be more efficiently softened by the 'Permutit' process, in which the water is filtered through zeolite (sodium aluminium silicate), or on a smaller scale by the use of a chemical called 'Calgon'.

## The Collection of Water

Water for a water-supply may be collected from rain, from surface water, or from ground water.

**Rain water** may be collected off roofs into barrels or tanks. It is soft, flat and contaminated with what it has absorbed from the atmosphere or from the roof. It is suitable for washing and cooking, but the impurities in it and its flatness make it unsuitable for drinking.

**Surface water** is collected in upland regions from streams, rivers and lakes. To provide a constant store of water a valley has to be dammed and a reservoir formed. From the reservoir water flows by gravity through aqueducts of cast-iron or concrete to underground reservoirs near the town it supplies. Good upland water is unpolluted and does not need bacterial purification. The upper reaches of rivers, above centres of population, are usually free from pollution. Lower reaches are usually contaminated by sewage, and water taken from them has to be purified before it can be used.

**Ground water** has soaked through the ground and been held up by an impervious layer. Where the impervious layer is in contact with the surface of the ground, as it may be on the slope of a hill, the water emerges as a spring. Small springs usually flow only in wet weather and dry up in dry weather. Main springs, from deeper sources and greater supplies of water, may be copious and unfailing.

*Wells* are sunk in order to tap ground water. They may be shallow, deep or artesian (see Fig. 11).

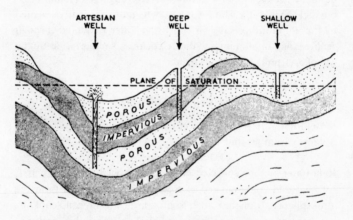

FIG. 11. *Diagram showing a shallow and deep well and an artesian well*

*Shallow wells* tap water above the first impervious layer; the nearer this layer is to the surface the more likely is the water to be polluted.

*Deep wells* tap water lying under the first impervious layer, the water having got there by percolation from higher ground. This water is usually pure, provided that the well is properly constructed of water-tight walls and that the water is pumped out of it and not drawn up in a bucket.

*Artesian wells* (called after the town of Artois in France) tap water at a still deeper level. In any porous ground the water will rise up to a level called the plane of saturation; and if an artesian well is sunk in a valley where the plane of saturation in the higher ground around is actually higher than the top of the well, water will gush out of the well without any pumping. Water from an artesian well is pure and hard.

Water is distributed to houses and buildings through iron pipes. To ensure that it reaches all buildings in a town, those on hills as well as those in valleys, pumps force the water through the pipes under pressure. A pressure of 40 lb. per square inch is sufficient for all ordinary purposes and for the fire services.

## Diseases spread by Water

Some diseases are easily spread by water, almost invariably by the water becoming contaminated by human faeces. These diseases include: typhoid fever, paratyphoid fever, dysentery, poliomyelitis, cholera, leptospira icterohaemorrhagica.

Lead poisoning has occurred as a result of drinking water having been passed through lead pipes.

*Bacteriological Testing.* Because of the great danger of serious disease being spread by water, all water used for domestic purposes should be regularly tested for bacteriological purity. It has been found that estimating the number of *Escherichia Coli* in the water is adequate to decide whether it has been contaminated by sewage. The best water contains no *E. Coli*; the presence of 1–2 bacilli in 100 ml of water is not regarded as dangerous; but the presence of more bacilli is suspicious of contamination.

## Purification of Water

Water from deep and artesian wells is usually pure. Water from uplands is usually pure if care is taken that the area is not contaminated. Water from shallow wells is often contaminated, especially if the people using it are careless about hygiene. Water from the lower reaches of rivers is almost always contaminated by sewage.

The purification of water is achieved mainly by three methods—by storage, by filtration, and by chemical action. The method used depends upon the source of the water and its degree of contamination as decided by bacteriological examination; where there is severe contamination several processes may be used in combination.

*Storage.* Water collected from uplands is stored in reservoirs (formed by damming a valley) or in natural lakes. Micro-organisms in it are exposed to the effects of sunlight, air, and other creatures in the water. Odours are discharged from the surface, impurities sink to the bottom, and the bacterial content is greatly reduced. Under such conditions any typhoid bacilli die within a month, most of them within a week.

*Filtration.* Filtration is the usual method of purification when water is likely to be contaminated, as, for instance, when it is drawn out of a river. The water is filtered through layers of sand and gravel, the bacteria being separated off with other forms of organic life in a film on the surface. This 'slow sand filtration' may not be quick enough where very large amounts of water are required; and there is a more rapid method in which the water passes through shallow basins in which the bacteria are precipitated, and then forced under pressure through sand and gravel. By this rapid method (which is about fifty times as fast as the slow method) about 125 million gallons of water can be purified for each acre of filter surface per day.

*Chemical Purification.* The usual method is by chlorine gas forced under pressure through the water, a method that can safely and rapidly purify heavily contaminated water. For clear water a dose of 0·1 part of chlorine per million of water is necessary; for water taken from the Thames above London 0·25–1·0 part per million is necessary.

In these ways water can be purified on a large scale. A nurse should know how small quantities of suspected water can be made safe for drinking. There are two easy ways:

1. *Boiling.* If water is boiled for five minutes, all dangerous micro-organisms are killed.

2. *Bleaching Powder.* Bleaching powder (chlorinated lime) con-

tains 33 per cent of available chlorine. To sterilize water, add half a teaspoonful of bleaching powder to one pint of water. From this pint of water take one teaspoonful and put this teaspoonful into ten gallons of water. In half an hour the water will be fit to drink.

## Protection of Water Supplies

One of the most important duties of a Regional Water Authority is to ensure that the water it supplies is protected from contamination. In addition to carrying out the appropriate methods of water purification, it has to take these precautions:

1. *The source of the water supply* must be kept under supervision. In the upland regions from which water is drawn, all houses must be fitted with proper sanitation, and no pollution of the water by manure must be allowed to occur. Rivers and streams from which water is drawn must be inspected for possible sources of contamination. Wells must have water-tight walls.

2. *Bacteriological examinations* of the water must be made at frequent intervals, and the water examined for chemical changes.

3. *Filtration and chlorination plants* must be adequately supervised.

4. *Repairs* to pipes and plants must be carefully supervised. No workman engaged in the water services must be allowed to defaecate underground, and adequate facilities must be available underground for micturition.

5. *Workmen* must be tested before they are engaged for the water services. Tests should be done on blood, urine and faeces for evidence of past typhoid and paratyphoid infection and for the detection of carriers. No man must be allowed to work if he has diarrhoea. Workmen should be instructed in hygienic practices and carefully supervised.

**Swimming Baths.** The water in a swimming bath should be up to the best bacteriological standards of drinking water—it should not contain *E. Coli*. As the water is likely to be contaminated from the bodies of bathers, it should be subjected to cleansing processes.

In modern swimming baths the water is in continuous circulation, so that all of it is passed through the cleansing apparatus every four hours (see Fig. 12). As it passes out of the bath, the water is passed through a screen to remove large objects, dosed with filter-alum and soda, passed under pressure through a filter, aerated, warmed if necessary, and chlorinated to 0·2–0·5 part of chlorine per million parts of the water, and then returned to the other end of the bath. Concentrations of chlorine above 0·5 part per million are not used because they make the bathers' eyes smart.

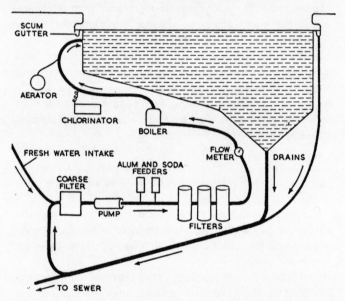

FIG. 12. *Circulation of water in a swimming bath*

Bathers should wash under a shower before entering the bath. To prevent infections of the feet by fungus infections, all surfaces on which the bathers tread should be hosed down frequently, and the bathers should be able to enter the bath only after walking through a shallow foot-bath containing hypochlorite solution. People with plantar warts or molluscum contagiosum, both contagious diseases due to infective agents, should not use public baths until they have been cured.

Adequate lavatory accommodation should be provided. The bath should have a channel round it into which the bather can spit. The sides and bottom of the bath should be kept clean and free from growths and deposits.

# Chapter Nine

# THE DISPOSAL OF REFUSE AND SEWAGE

## Dry Refuse

A thousand people produce about a ton of rubbish a day, and disposing of tons of refuse is a major problem of local authorities. The refuse consists of ashes, paper, cardboard, tins, broken glass and crockery, old boxes, unwanted furniture and kitchen waste. Hospitals turn out dirty dressings and old plasters as well as ordinary refuse.

As much as possible of the refuse should be burned, either on domestic fires or in incinerators. What cannot be burned should be kept in dustbins. Waste paper can be collected in sacks. A dustbin should have a well-fitting lid, which should be kept on. Dustbins are usually emptied by the local authority's refuse-collectors at weekly intervals. In country districts refuse is usually tipped into ash-pits, which are emptied from time to time.

The *Garcey system* is used in blocks of flats. Each flat has a water-flushed chute for refuse, which falls to a collecting-station in the basement, where the water is removed and the refuse incinerated.

*Garbage grinders* can be attached to a kitchen sink and used to cut up organic matter (e.g. potato peelings), which is then passed into the sewage system. It cannot be used for other refuse.

**Disposal by Local Authority.** The local authority may dispose of the refuse in several ways.

*Sorting.* The refuse may be sorted for objects that can be sold, such as tins and bottles.

*Incineration.* The burnable rubbish is burned in an incinerator. The furnace clinker produced may be sold for making concrete.

*Regulated tipping* (Controlled tipping). The rubbish is spread on waste land in layers 5 feet thick; each layer of rubbish is covered by a layer of earth 1 foot thick; and each layer is allowed to settle before being covered by another layer. The ground is sprayed with D.D.T. or other insecticide to kill flies, and the area is surrounded by wire netting to keep out rats and dogs. Low-lying land is usually used.

*Disposal by Sea.* Refuse may be disposed of in the sea by being taken out in barges and dumped out to sea on the ebb-tide so far out that it is not brought back by the tides.

## Sewage

Sewage is composed of:
    human excreta
    waste water from houses and factories
    rain water
There are three main ways of removing it.

The *Combined System* is usual in towns and cities: it takes all sewage.

The *Separate System* takes human excreta and waste water in one set of pipes and rain water in another.

The *Conservancy System* is used in a few country districts: the excreta are passed into a pail in a privy. The pail is emptied at least once a week but preferably oftener and the contents are buried. A privy should be out of doors and at least 6 feet from a house and 40 feet from a well or spring. Chemical privies can be obtained in which the excreta are treated with a disinfectant. In country houses with a piped water supply, the excreta and waste water flow into a cess-pool, which is periodically emptied. Where no cess-pool is available, house waste water is run into a pit or sedimentation tank with an overflow into a stream or drain.

## The Combined System of Sewage Disposal

*1. Human Excreta.* The water-closet should be made in one piece of glazed stoneware, fireclay or porcelain. The seat should be hinged. In public lavatories, where standards of hygiene may not be high, the seat should have a gap in front. The water cistern should discharge 2–3 gallons at a time and flush the water-closet

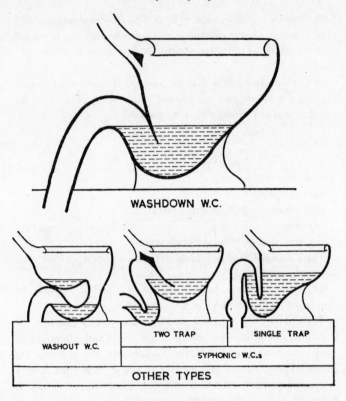

WASHDOWN W.C.

| WASHOUT W.C. | TWO TRAP | SINGLE TRAP |
| | SYPHONIC W.C.s | |
| OTHER TYPES | | |

FIG. 13. *Diagram showing a modern washdown W.C. and three obsolete types*

round the rim and so clean the pan (see Fig. 13). The lavatory should have at least one outside wall with a window in it. The pipe from the w.c. is called the soil-pipe. At the bottom of the w.c. or in the first part of the soil-pipe there must be a P or S trap. A trap is a bend that holds water, ensuring that there is always some water between the w.c. and the drainage system and preventing gases from entering the lavatory from the pipes.

The soil-pipe is made of iron or plastic, has water-tight joints, and enters directly into the house-drain. Where water-closets are arranged one above another on different floors, an extension of the soil-pipe is carried vertically up to the roof where it opens, away from windows and chimneys, and ventilates the pipe.

Urinals and hospital slop-sinks should be 'trapped' like water-closets.

*2. House Waste Water.* Baths, sinks and wash-basins are usually made of vitrified earthenware. They should be 'trapped' by P or S traps fitted with a screw that can be unscrewed for cleaning the trap when it becomes blocked (see Fig. 14). The water flows through a waste-pipe, 2 in (5 cm) in diameter, directly into the house-drain. Where a series of basins, sinks or baths are arranged to discharge waste at different floors into the same waste-pipe, the pipe should be extended up to the roof for ventilation.

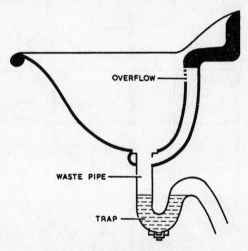

FIG. 14. *Washbasin with drain*

The waste water from the kitchens of hospitals and other institutions should open into a stoneware 'grease gully' (where grease in the water will settle out) before passing through a trap into the waste-pipe. The grease gully should be cleaned out two or three times a week.

*3. Rain Water* is collected into gutters, runs down the rain-pipes, and goes through underground P or S traps into the house-drain.

*4. House-Drains* take the waste from soil-pipes, waste-pipes and rain-pipes. They are made of glazed fireclay, stoneware or cast iron. The drain runs downwards to the sewer, and the narrower the drain the steeper must be the fall. There should be a trap between sewer and drain to prevent the entry of sewer gases into the drain (see Fig. 15).

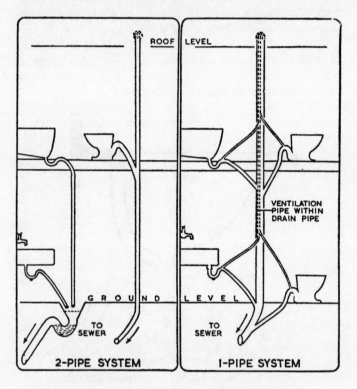

FIG. 15. *Diagram of the side of a house with drainpipe*

*5. Sewers* are large pipes usually made of concrete. They are placed under roads and as far as possible in straight lines. They have man-holes at intervals through which men can get into the sewers to inspect and clean them. They are ventilated by shafts opening at road level or occasionally carried up above the roofs of houses. A sewer must 'fall' (run downwards); and the size and fall of the sewer must be sufficient to take off domestic waste water, industrial waste water, and the large amounts of rain water that may flow into the system during a storm.

Sewer-men, whose job is to inspect and clean sewers, run several risks: of being drowned by flood-water during storms, of being gassed by gas from a leaking main, of being killed by petrol getting into a sewer and exploding, of being infected with *Leptospira ictero-haemorrhagica*.

Sewers may run into:

(a) a sewage works;

(b) a river after some purification;

(c) the sea—a common method of disposal at seaside towns; although the sewage is discharged below low-water and when the tide is ebbing, the next tide may bring it back or deposit it on the beach of some other seaside town. Bathing in sewage-contaminated sea water may be unpleasant.

6. *Sewage Works.* Sewage is heavily contaminated with *E. Coli* (to the extent of 100,000 organisms per ml) and other organisms. A sewage works has to remove solid matter from the sewage and reduce its bacterial content to a safe level. However clean the effluent from the sewage works, any river it passes into is regarded as sewage-polluted and its water as unfit to drink without further treatment (see Water Supplies). The modern use of detergents in washing has produced a new problem—the production of huge masses of foam at sewage works and on the surfaces of rivers into which the effluent has passed.

Sewage purification depends upon the joint use of (a) Preliminary Processes and (b) Completing Processes.

(a) *Preliminary Processes* are designed to remove gross matter and solids suspended in the sewage. *Screening* through bars or on an endless moving-belt of wire-mesh removes the gross matter. After screening the sewage passes into a *grit-chamber*, where heavy particles settle. Thence it passes into a *continuous flow sedimentation tank*; its flow through this tank is slow, suspended matter sinks as a deposit (called sludge), and from the floor the sludge is removed every few days. Some authorities purify the sewage and recover annually thousands of tons of sludge-fertilizer for use on farms.

(b) *Completing Processes* are designed to break down the remaining nitrogenous matter into simple substances and remove organisms. Animal protein deposited in soil begins to disintegrate at once, under the actions of enzymes and bacteria; faeces and urine are broken down to ammonia; and in the soil the ammonia is converted into nitrates, which are absorbed by plants. The completing process is carried out in one of three ways: Land Treatment, Filtration and Bio-aeration.

*1. Land Treatment.* The sewage is distributed by gravity over the soil of a *sewage-farm*, on which crops can be grown. Sewage-farms are efficient purifiers of sewage, but they require much land, which is not always available.

*2. Filtration Method.* The sewage is filtered through beds of clinker (e.g. by the revolving arms seen at many sewage-works); a gelatinous film of bacteria is formed on the clinker, the film absorbs oxygen from the air, and the organic matter is broken down by bacterial action into carbon dioxide, nitrogen and other simple chemical substances.

*3. Bio-Aeration* (Activated Sludge Process). The sewage is agitated continuously by paddles or compressed air; particles separate out, develop biological properties, and purify the sewage.

# Chapter Ten

# PETS, PESTS AND VERMIN

## Pets

**Cats and Dogs.** The extent to which cats and dogs can be a danger to health is little appreciated in Britain. Both animals can spread diseases. Cats and dogs can be infected by the salmonella organisms; in Britain between 1 and 2 per cent of them are infected and in the U.S.A. over 27 per cent, and human beings can become infected by direct handling or from faecally-contaminated dust.

The common roundworm of dog, and possibly the common roundworm of cat, may be harmful to man. Infection again is via the animal's faeces, and the larvae, wandering through the human body, are liable to produce infection, pulmonary infiltrations, epilepsy (by invading the brain) and endophthalmitis (by invading the eye).

Cats may also infect man with ringworm and cat-scratch fever, and dogs infect him with ringworm, rabies and hydatid disease. In countries such as Australia where animals are commonly infested with the dog tapeworm and the hydatid tapeworm, special precautions have to be taken, the animals being dewormed, being kept away from children, and their coats being disinfected by insecticides. Rabies, a virus infection of animals, liable to be contracted by man from the bite of an infected dog, is prevented in Britain by the strict quarantining of all dogs, and other animals likely to carry the disease, brought into the country from abroad.

It is obviously impossible to prevent children from fondling their pets, but they should be encouraged to wash their hands after fondling their animals and before eating. Dogs should not be allowed to lick children's faces and hands. Dogs and cats should not be allowed to be where food is prepared and should be banned from food shops.

**Birds.** Psittacosis is a disease that can be transmitted to man from birds. It is a virus infection which produces in man a severe atypical haemorrhagic pneumonia, the mortality from which was at one time very high. Man is infected by direct contact with a sick bird or by the inhalation of infected dust. Birds that commonly develop the disease are the parrot (especially the green Amazon parrot), the budgerigar, the canary and the pigeon. The forbidding of the importation of the parrot into this country was followed by a reduction in the incidence of the disease. The prevention of the disease is by the destruction of sick birds, discouragement of the fondling of sick birds, and the keeping of scrupulously clean cages.

Birdfancier's disease is an allergic reaction to the inhalation of dust from bird-droppings or feathers and repeated attacks of this pneumonia-like illness can cause fibrosis of the lungs.

**Other Pets.** *Tortoises* are often heavily infected with salmonella organisms and so are a cause of food poisoning. *Monkeys* can spread virus infection which, relatively mild in the monkey, can be fatal to man. Tortoises and monkeys should not be kept as pets; they are too dangerous.

## Pests

**The House Fly.** House flies are prevalent during the late summer. Each female can lay between 600 and 900 eggs and lays them for preference in horse manure or decaying vegetable matter. Flies survive the winter by staying in a warm place and larvae or pupae lie dormant until summer (see Fig. 16).

House flies like to feed on human faeces or on human food such as milk, jam, sugar and butter, often flying straight from faeces to food. They can spread both infectious micro-organisms and the eggs of parasitic worms, by excreting them or by spreading them with their mouths, legs and bodies. In this country they are often responsible for attacks of 'summer diarrhoea' in children and are particularly dangerous in country districts. In tropical countries they are responsible for much cholera, dysentery, typhoid fever and worm infestation.

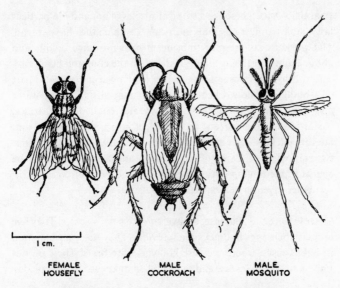

1 cm.

FEMALE        MALE        MALE.
HOUSEFLY     COCKROACH   MOSQUITO

FIG. 16. *Housefly, cockroach and mosquito*

They may be killed by D.D.T., pyrethrum sprays or other insecticides. Unfortunately the use of one of these insecticides is usually followed by the appearance of 'resistant' strains—insects on which that particular insecticide has no effect. These resistant strains are probably ones descended from flies that are for some reason not affected by that particular insecticide; while the other flies are killed off, these resistant strains can live and breed.

**The Cockroach.** There are two kinds of cockroach (black-beetle) in this country, one about an inch long (2·5 cm) and the other about half the size. They hide in cracks, especially where there is some heat—as, for instance, behind heating pipes—and come out at night. They foul food with their excreta, but are not known to spread any disease.

They may be killed by D.D.T., pyrethrum, powdered borax and sodium fluoride. The holes by which they get into a room should if possible be blocked up with cement.

**Pharaoh's Ants.** These are a tropical species of ant and are particularly liable to infect hospitals in Britain, to which they have spread. The worker ants are of a translucent brown-orange colour and about 2 mm long (being much smaller than the common black ant). The ants live in thousands in colonies in any warm, concealed part of a building. The workers forage over long distances for water and food; they have a liking for raw and cooked meat, trifles, custards and other sweets. They can get into beds, dressings and laundry packets. They can be infected with many micro-organisms, e.g. staphylococci, streptococci, *E. coli*, and are suspected to be agents in continuing infections in hospitals. Prevention is by insecticides given under expert advice.

**Silver fish** are tiny, flat insects covered with silvery scales. They live and lay their eggs in cracks and crevices. They are very common in bakehouses, where they are known as fire-brats. They are not known to spread disease and can be killed by the usual insecticides.

### Vermin

**Rats.** The black rat and the brown rat are the two kinds found in Great Britain. They are distinguishable not so much by their colour, which is variable, as by their habits. The black rat was originally a native of the tropics and lived in trees; it retains an arboreal habit of getting about, climbing into buildings through windows and skylights and moving from building to building by running along overhead cables; and, being originally a tropical animal, it has in cold countries to live in houses or other buildings. The brown rat is a native of northern Europe and Asia, goes about on land, swims strongly, gets into buildings via sewers and drains, is more robust than the black rat (which it kills or drives away when they meet), and can survive in the open.

Female rats breed from the age of six months and produce litters of about eight young four or five times a year. The rat population of Britain has been estimated to be about equal to the human population.

Rats do an enormous amount of damage. They eat grain, root

crops, fruit and vegetables, consuming or damaging about 10 per cent of the world's food. They kill and eat poultry and game. They destroy woodwork, strip insulating materials off electric wires, perforate pipes, and tear up clothing for nesting materials. Both the black and the brown rat can be carriers of plague-infected fleas, which spread epidemics of plague among rats and men. About half the rats in Britain are infected with the spirochetes of Weil's disease and rat-bite fever.

*Prevention of Rat Infestation*

1. Buildings and ships should be constructed in such ways that rats cannot easily enter them or find nesting-places.

2. Buildings should be 'ratproofed' by wire mesh so that rats cannot get in through drains, cellars, windows, sky-lights, etc.

3. Rats should be killed by traps and poisoned baits or by fumigation with lethal gases.

4. Rats should be prevented from getting on or off ships.

5. Garbage should not be allowed to accumulate near buildings: dustbins should be of metal and have closely-fitting lids.

6. Cats keep down rats on farms, but they are not much use in buildings where they cannot get into places rats live in and in foodshops are a danger to human health.

*Destruction.* Warfarin is the drug usually used to kills rats. It is an anticoagulant which blocks vitamin K metabolism and so stops blood from clotting. In many areas of Britain rats have become resistant to it, and where this has happened a combination of warfarin with vitamin D is used, rats which eat it dying of too little vitamin K and too much vitamin D. Other, more dangerous drugs can be used in special circumstances, but they are too dangerous to be used generally.

**Mice** are mature at three months and produce several litters a year. They destroy woodwork and fabrics, but do much less damage than rats. They foul food and contaminate it with food-poisoning micro-organisms. Their numbers can be kept down by cats, traps and poisoned baits.

# Chapter Eleven

# PARASITES

Parasites are creatures that live in or on the bodies of other creatures and do them harm. In tropical countries they are a common cause of serious human illness, but in the colder climate of Britain, with its high standards of hygiene, they cause much less illness. Precautions must, however, be taken, and there is always a danger that travellers will bring to this country a parasite that does not normally live here. Parasites may be external (living on or in the skin) or internal (living in the body).

*External Parasites.* Lice, Fleas, Scabies Mite, Bedbugs.

*Internal Parasites.* Threadworms, Tapeworms, Roundworms, Trichomonas vaginalis, Malaria parasite, Toxoplasmosis.

## External Parasites

**1. Lice.** Man can be infected by three kinds of lice: the Head Louse, the Body Louse and the Pubic Louse (see Fig. 17).

Lice are little flat insects. They have six legs with which to scuttle over the skin, and on the end of each leg a little claw for holding on to hair with. Lice are 'selective' insects: that means they can live only on one kind of host; human lice, for instance, can only live on human beings, dog lice only on dogs. They live by sucking the blood of their host and have a life of four to six weeks. They breed by laying eggs called 'nits', which hatch out directly into little lice.

The human *Head Louse* lives in the hair of the scalp and beard. It is from 1 to 2 millimetres long, and so is large enough to be seen by the naked eye. Its greyish-white body is easily seen in dark hair, but not so easily in light or white hair. Its nits are white and stick to the hair; they can be distinguished from pieces of scurf by not coming off the hair when it is lightly run through the fingers.

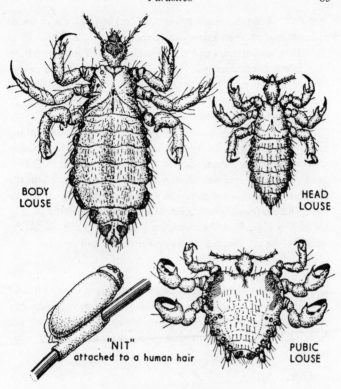

BODY
LOUSE

HEAD
LOUSE

"NIT"
attached to a human hair

PUBIC
LOUSE

FIG. 17. *Three varieties of louse and a nit*
(*greatly magnified*)

In her lifetime the female lays about 100 nits. Although infestation
of the hair of school children has disappeared from many parts
of Britain, it is still a serious problem in many overcrowded industrial areas.

The human *Body Louse* is larger than the head louse, lays two
or three times as many eggs, and lays them, not in the hair, but
in the creases of clothing and bedclothing.

The *Pubic* or *Crab Louse* is smaller than the other lice. It lives
in the pubic hair, to which it attaches its eggs, and sometimes in
other hairy parts. It is not known to spread any disease.

Body lice (and to a lesser extent head lice) spread these diseases: endemic typhus fever, European relapsing fever.

An itchy spot appears where a louse has bitten. People who have been infested for years may not feel any discomfort, but newly-infested people may be severely irritated. People are liable to infect themselves by rubbing into a scratch the excreta or body of a louse dead of one of these diseases.

Infestation can be prevented by cleanliness of body and clothing and by avoiding crowds. The lice can be killed by D.D.T., Gammexane and other insecticides. A 2 per cent emulsion of D.D.T. or of gamma benzene hexachloride, rubbed into the hair kills the lice and lasts long enough to kill young lice hatching out of the eggs. The treatment is best given as a shampoo, repeated once at the end of a week. All infested members of a family should be treated at the same time. Lice, like other insects, can develop resistance to insecticides.

**2. Fleas** are tiny insects with bodies flattened from side to side and legs adapted for jumping (see Fig. 18). The common human flea can jump a foot in distance and 8 inches in height. They are not 'selective': they do not mind what species of animal they are living on.

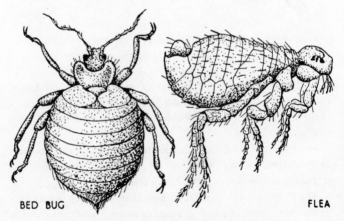

BED BUG      FLEA

Fig. 18. *Bedbug and flea (greatly magnified)*

*Pulex irritans* is the common human flea. It lives for a year, feeds on blood (but can go for three or four months without a meal), and lays its eggs in the cracks of floors and furniture. The egg turns into a larva and the larva into a pupa (chrysalis), which can stay in that state for a year if conditions are not right for it to develop into a flea. It lives equally well on men, dogs, rats, mice, pigs and cattle. Where it bites, it causes itching or a red papule; some people develop urticarial swellings around the bites.

It can spread the following diseases:

bubonic plague

anthrax

infestation by the dog tapeworm

*Plague fleas* are more serious. Normally they live on rats, and by biting rats infected with plague become carriers of the plague bacillus. An epidemic of plague among rats causes them to die in large numbers, and when this happens the fleas transfer themselves to men, bite them and infect them with plague. Plague, the Black Death of the Middle Ages, stills occurs in the East.

Destruction of rats is the main preventive measure. The fleas can be killed by D.D.T. and other insecticides.

**3. Scabies Mite.** Scabies is spread by a small semi-transparent insect called a mite. The female of the species is chiefly responsible for the symptoms of the disease, and an infected person usually has about a dozen on him. The female mites can burrow in the skin at the rate of about 5 millimetres a day, and as they advance they lay their eggs in the burrow behind them. The eggs hatch out into larvae, which in their turn make new burrows. Young male

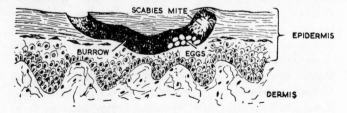

FIG. 19. *Scabies mite laying eggs in burrow*

and female mites are formed from the larvae, and the males come out on to the surface of the skin to hunt for the females. Norwegian or crusted scabies is a rare but very infectious form of scabies, in which the skin swarms with mites; if unrecognized and untreated it is liable to cause epidemics of scabies in small communities, such as a children's home.

The common symptoms are an intense itching and an inflammation of the skin, which is scratched and secondarily infected. Transmission is by direct contact between people. Treatment is by the application of gamma benzene hexachloride, monosulfiram, etc.

**4. Bedbugs.** A bedbug is a small insect with an oval, flat body and six legs. By day it hides in cracks and crevices in walls and furniture or under wallpaper; by night it comes out to suck blood from man. It is a common inhabitant of slums. Usually it feeds on blood every second or third night, but it can live for a year without a feed. In cold weather it hibernates. It is not known to transmit any disease, but its bites cause much irritation and loss of sleep.

Getting rid of bedbugs from a house was formerly a major operation undertaken by the local health authority and involved the tearing out and burning of much woodwork. Bedbugs are now killed by insecticides. It is important that infected furniture be treated before it is moved to a new house.

### Internal Parasites

**1. Threadworms** are thin, little white worms, which live in large numbers in the caecum and appendix of their host (see Fig. 20). Man is their only host, and they occur most commonly in children. The females are longer and more numerous than the males. After fertilization they move along the colon and out of the anus to lay their eggs on the outside of the body, usually in the perianal region or on the buttocks. The eggs are sticky and stay where they are laid. In warm, moist conditions the larvae in them can survive for several weeks; but in the air, in dust and with exposure to sunshine, they die in a few days. In suspected cases, when the worm cannot be found, eggs may be found by pressing a piece of sticky

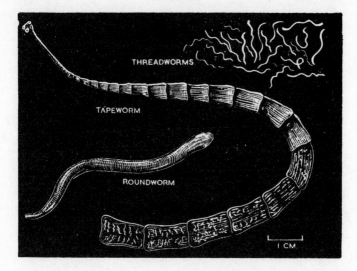

FIG. 20. *Threadworm, roundworm and tapeworm*

cellulose tape over the anal region and examining it under a microscope.

Man is infected by swallowing the eggs. An already infected person can be reinfected by: (a) contaminating his fingers with the eggs from his own perianal region and transferring them to his mouth; and (b) the eggs hatching out in the perianal region and the larvae crawling back up the anus into the colon. Other people can be infected by: (a) contaminating their fingers with the eggs; (b) becoming infected from lavatory seats; and (c) by swallowing eggs shaken out of clothes and bedclothes. It is common to find several members of a family infected.

*Prevention* is by:

1. Careful washing of the anal region and hands after having the bowels open.

2. Frequent washing of bedclothes and underclothes and the exposure of them to wind and sun.

3. Cleanliness of lavatory seats.

*Treatment* is by piperazine citrate or viprynium.

**2. Tapeworms.** The only common tapeworm in this country is the *Beef Tapeworm*. It is so called because for part of its life-cycle it has to live in cattle.

In human beings it lives in the small intestine. It can grow to a length of 40 feet (12 metres) and 2,000 segments, and can live for ten years.

A tapeworm consists of a head, a neck and a chain of segments (see Fig. 20). The head is very small, compared with the size of the segments and the length of the worm; it sticks to the mucous membrane of the small intestine by means of suckers. It has no mouth and absorbs its food directly through the walls of its segments from the intestinal contents in which it lives. The neck is the region of growth from which each segment is formed; and as each is formed it pushes away the segment that has been formed just before it. The segments are small at first, but get larger as they grow older and farther away from the neck. Each segment contains male and female organs; fertilized eggs are formed in the segment, which becomes detached from the worm, degenerates and discharges its eggs. Usually only one worm is present at a time; its presence seems to prevent other worms from growing. It may not cause any symptoms other than vague abdominal disturbance, and the appearance of segments at the anus may be the first sign of its presence. They are discharged with the faeces or wriggle out to deposit their eggs on the clothes or bedclothes.

The eggs die unless they are eaten by cattle, which can happen when cattle graze pastures infected with human faeces or sewage. Once swallowed, the embryos appear from the eggs, pass through the intestinal wall, invade the tissues and settle down in striped muscle, where each embryo forms a small cyst (called a cysticercus or bladderworm) containing a tapeworm head. The muscles usually affected are those of the heart, jaw, tongue and diaphragm. Nothing further happens unless the beef is eaten by a man with the cyst intact. This means that the beef must be eaten raw or imperfectly cooked. The cyst is then digested in the man's intestine, the head appears and attaches itself to the mucous membrane, and another worm starts to grow.

*Treatment* is by niclosamide or mepacrine hydrochloride.

Other tapeworms that may infest man are the *Pork Tapeworm* (which spends part of its life in the pig, causes pork to appear 'measly', and is capable of forming small cysts in human tissues as well as living in the intestine); the *Fish Tapeworm* (which spends part of its life in freshwater fish); the *Dog Tapeworm* (which spends part of its life in a dog flea); and the *Hydatid Tapeworm* (which spends part of its life in a dog, cat or other animal, and is liable to produce in man large cysts).

*Prevention of All Kinds of Tapeworm Infection*

1. Abstinence from eating raw or imperfectly-cooked beef, pork or freshwater fish.

2. Sanitary disposal of human excreta.

3. Careful personal and community hygiene.

4. Thorough meat inspection.

5. Special precautions where dogs are involved, e.g. disinfestation by D.D.T., deworming, care that dogs cannot get near food, crockery and children.

## 3. Roundworms

(a) *Ascaris lumbricoides.* This roundworm lives only in man. It is 6 to 12 inches (15 to 30 cm) long, and can live for a year in a man's intestine. He may be infected by many worms at one time; sometimes masses of them will cause intestinal obstruction or one of them get into his bile-duct or appendix. The eggs pass out of the anus. They are very resistant: in damp earth they can live for at least five years, ordinary sewage treatment does not always kill them, and antiseptics in the concentrations normally used have little effect upon them. Infection of man is through his mouth. The embryos follow a peculiar course. They bore through the wall of the intestine and into the veins, go round in the blood to the right side of the heart and the lungs; they crawl out of the lungs, up the trachea and larynx, and then down the oesophagus into the stomach and small intestine (where they started from) to turn into adult worms.

*Treatment* is by piperazine phosphate or bephenium.

*Prevention* is by careful hygiene, the sanitary disposal of human excreta, training of children not to eat sweets that have dropped to the ground, and treatment of infected soil by deep burial or exposure to steam.

(*Ascaris* in pigs is not a danger as the human and pig strains are quite different.)

(b) *Trichiniasis* (Trichinosis). Trichiniasis is infection by the round-worm Trichinella spiralis. Man is usually infected by eating the raw or partly-cooked flesh of pigs, which have themselves been infected by eating infected rats or other animals. A common source of infection is sausage-meat, which some children like to eat raw. Infected pork is called 'measly', but this name is also given to pork infected with pork tapeworm.

Adult worms are 2–4 mm long and live as parasites in the intestine. Their larvae invade the lymphatics of the intestine and are distributed all over the body in the blood-stream. In muscle the larvae form cysts, which ultimately become calcified. The parasite does not spread directly from man to man.

*Treatment:* piperazine phosphate or bephenium hydroxynaphthoate.

*Prevention:* abstinence from eating raw pig meat; pig meat to be cooked to at least 140° F (60° C) for at least 30 minutes per pound so that all the meat is cooked and not only the outside; freezing of pork at 0° F (32° C) for at least 24 hours; thorough meat inspection.

**4. The Whipworm** is common in the tropics and other warm countries and may be brought to Britain by immigrants. Children are particularly liable to be infected. The worm is whip-shaped and 30–50 mm long.

It lives in the large intestine, and its eggs are excreted in the faeces. If the eggs are swallowed, the larvae hatch out and develop into adult worms, which attach themselves to the mucous membrane of the intestine. They can produce dysenteric symptoms and rectal prolapse. The diagnosis is made by recognition of the typical eggs in the faeces.

Bephenium hydroxynaphthoate and other anthelmintics can be tried.

**5. The Hookworm** is a common tropical infection. There are two varieties, the *Ankylostoma duodenale* and the *Necator americanus*. The adult worms attach themselves by their hooks to the wall of the small intestine, their eggs being excreted in the faeces. In suitable warm, moist conditions the larvae hatch out of the eggs and infect a new person by invading his skin. People particularly liable to be infected are those who walk barefoot or handle faecally contaminated soil. Having invaded the body, the larvae get into the circulation and reach the lungs; they pass out of the lungs up the trachea and reach the small intestine by passing down the oesophagus and through the stomach. Common evidence of infection are a severe hypochromic microcytic anaemia, malnutrition, and itching at the site of invasion of the skin. The diagnosis is made by finding the typical eggs in the faeces.

*Treatment* is by chenopodium, tetrachloroethylene or bephenium hydroxynaphthoate.

**6. The Malaria Parasite.** The parasite of malaria is a single-celled protozoon called Plasmodium. Four species of it can cause the disease:

*Plasmodium vivax:* causing a mild malaria, with bouts of fever typically every third day.

*Plasmodium falciparum:* causing the severe malignant malaria.

*Plasmodium malariae:* causing a mild but often chronic malaria.

*Plasmodium ovale:* causing a mild malaria.

The malaria parasite has two hosts: man and certain kinds of the Anopheles mosquito (see Fig. 16, page 79). The parasite has to live all its life in man or mosquito and cannot survive outside them. In its life-cycle the following events have to take place:

1. An infected mosquito has to bite a man and infect him with the malaria parasite.

2. The parasites have to multiply in the man and give him malaria.

3. Another mosquito has to bite the man and in turn become infected.

In the mosquito the parasites live in the salivary glands and are injected thousands at a time into man as the mosquito sucks blood from him. In man the parasites invade first the liver, where they multiply into many more thousands, and then into the red blood cells, where they multiply further. Each infected red blood cell is in time destroyed and more parasites are discharged into the bloodstream to attack more red blood cells.

The disease is now uncommon in Britain. Although by intensive efforts it has been abolished from many parts of the world (e.g. from Cyprus), it is still the greatest single cause of death, disease, malnutrition and chronic ill health in the world.

*Treatment:* Attacks of malaria in man are treated by various drugs, e.g. chloroquine, proguanil, amodiaquine, pyrimethamine.

*Prevention:*

1. *Attack on the Mosquito:* by spraying houses, buildings, ships, cars, trains and aeroplanes with insecticides such as D.D.T., B.H.C. (benzene hexachloride), Gammexane. Unfortunately 'resistant strains' of the mosquito appear that are not affected by the insecticide used.

2. *Attack on the Larva of the Mosquito:* the larvae live in still fresh water; their numbers may be reduced by draining marshy ground and spreading oil on the surface of the water and so preventing the larvae getting oxygen necessary for their life.

3. *Protection of Man from Mosquito:* building houses away from marshy ground; protection of windows with mosquito-proof wire-netting; covering exposed parts of the body after nightfall; sleeping under mosquito-netting.

4. *Improvement of Nutrition and General Health* of people living in malarious parts of the world.

**7. Trichomonas vaginalis** is a pear-shaped microscopic organism that may infect the vagina, causing a low-grade inflammation and a discharge. It can also occur in the genito-urinary tract of men. It does not form cysts. Spread of infection is possibly by sexual intercourse or from recently infected lavatory seats. Outside the body it does not live for long.

*Prevention:* by abstinence from promiscuous sexual intercourse; by thorough cleaning of lavatory seats; by the provision of lavatory seats with a gap in front.

*Treatment:* metronidazole by mouth.

**8. Toxoplasmosis.** Toxoplasma organisms are microscopic oval protoplasmic cells, occurring singly or in clusters. Infection by them seems to be becoming more common. Their life-cycle is unknown; birds and any warm-blooded animals can be infected. There is little positive evidence about the way in which the parasite is transmitted.

In humans the disease may occur as (a) an intra-uterine infection, (b) an early postnatal infection or (c) an infection of older children or adults. In England about 30 per cent of people are found to have been infected when special antibody tests are carried out on the blood, but clinical evidence of infection is rare. The organisms occur in many parts of the body, especially in nerves, muscles and capillary walls. They produce inflammatory changes and ultimately small areas of calcification. As an intra-uterine disease it may produce encephalitis, hydrocephalus, impaired vision and mental retardation. As a post-uterine disease it produces inflammatory changes, especially severe in lungs and kidneys.

The recommended treatment is a combination of sulphanilamide and pyrimethamine.

## Chapter Twelve

# ACCIDENTS IN THE HOME

Accidents in the home are second only to road accidents as the most common type of accident. If we take the average number of accidental deaths in Great Britain a day, we find they occur:

| | |
|---|---|
| In the home | 17 |
| On the road | 21 |
| At work | 2 |
| By train, water and air | 1 |
| By all other causes | 10 |

In Great Britain over 6,000 people are killed every year by accidents in the home, compared with over 7,500 deaths from road accidents. Moreover, from these accidents in the home, out of a population of about 54 million people, 80,000 are admitted into hospital every year, about $1\frac{1}{2}$ million attend out-patient departments, and an unknown number are treated for minor injuries by their own doctors, by district nurses or by first-aid organizations. Some of the injuries may be extremely severe; a badly-burnt child may have to spend over a year in hospital and may require, in the first desperate days, the attention of three or four doctors and five or six nurses.

Moreover, the victim of an accident, though his life be saved, may be maimed, permanently disfigured or profoundly disturbed psychologically.

The prevention of domestic accidents is therefore an important aspect of hygiene; and the kinds of accidents that happen in a home may very well happen in hospital to patient or nurse.

People of any age can suffer an accident at home, but two groups are particularly liable:

(a) Children under 5 years of age.

(b) People over 65.

The most common causes of accidents are *falls*, *burns* and *scalds*, *poisoning* and *suffocation*, as will be seen below.

## Home Accidents: Deaths in Great Britain
## for the year 1972

| Cause of Death | Age Groups (years) | | | | | Total |
|---|---|---|---|---|---|---|
| | 0–4 | 5–14 | 15–44 | 45–64 | 65 & over | |
| Falls | 57 | 14 | 99 | 327 | 3,740 | 4,237 |
| Poisoning | 18 | 10 | 228 | 262 | 185 | 703 |
| Burns and Scalds | 133 | 42 | 76 | 133 | 480 | 864 |
| Suffocation and Choking | 310 | 27 | 90 | 116 | 87 | 630 |
| Others | 102 | 17 | 67 | 68 | 150 | 404 |
| Total | 620 | 110 | 560 | 906 | 4,642 | 6,838 |

It will be seen from these figures that some groups are exposed to particular dangers:

*Children under 5* to suffocation, burns and scalds;

*Adults* to accidental poisoning;

*Old people* to falls, poisoning, burns and scalds.

**The Causes of Accidents.** An accident happens suddenly, without warning, and often only once in a lifetime. Some may be genuine accidents that could not have been anticipated or prevented; but most are the result of several factors acting together at the same time. There are two main factors:

(1) the *Human Factor*—the age, ignorance, carelessness or physical disability of the victim or of the person looking after the person who becomes a victim; and

(2) the *Material Factor*—the fault in the home where the accident happens. One can see a combination of several factors in this kind of accident: a toddler (human element) is left alone by her mother (human element) and sets her highly-inflammable nightie (physical factor) on fire at an unguarded fire (physical factor).

Among the *human factors* are such things as:

(a) overcrowding;

(b) married women going out to work, coming home tired, and giving less supervision to children and help to the old;

(c) children being ignorant, curious, wilful, disobedient, or (as toddlers) badly co-ordinated in their movements;

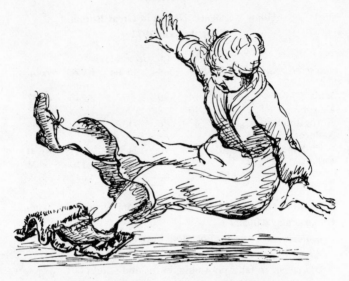

FIG. 21. *Old woman falling on a loose rug*

(d) adults being worried, hurried, tired, depressed, careless or negligent;

(e) old people living alone, being obstinate, forgetful and neglectful;

(f) such physical conditions as epilepsy, spastic paralysis, fainting attacks, dizziness, tottering gait, arteriosclerosis, impaired sight, hearing and smell.

*Falls* may be due to:

(a) badly-designed houses, poor lighting, slippery floors, loose rugs, holes in carpets and lino, loose stair-rods, spilt grease, obstacles left lying on the floor or stairs, unguarded windows, high prams and cots with inadequate safety-harness; and (b) hurry, wearing unsuitable shoes, trying to manage without a light, standing on rickety chairs and steps, over-reaching (see Fig. 21).

*Burns* may be caused by:

(a) contact of clothes with an unguarded fire—coal, electric, gas or oil;

(b) wearing inflammable clothes, especially dresses or nighties of winceyette and flannelette; wearing nighties (which cause about twenty-three times as many deaths as pyjamas); cotton saris worn by Indian women catch fire very easily;

(c) falling against the bars of a coal fire or grasping the element of an electric fire;

(d) using inflammable cleaning solvents indoors near naked lights;

(e) pouring methylated spirits or paraffin to get a fire to burn;

(f) electric blankets setting bedclothes on fire.

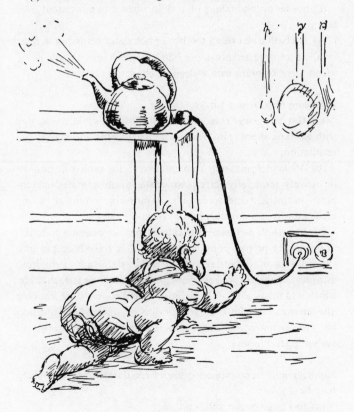

FIG. 22. *Child crawling and pulling on an electric kettle flex*

*Scalds* may be caused by:

(a) a child reaching for a cup only just within reach;

(b) a child upsetting a saucepan whose handle is sticking outwards from the stove;

(c) a child pulling on the dangling loop of flex to an electric kettle (see Fig. 22);

(d) a child pulling on the table-cloth and upsetting the teapot, or jerking his mother's arm as she pours out;

(e) a child coming into contact with steam from the outward-turned spout of a kettle;

(f) hot fat or fluid falling on a child when a pan is passed over him;

(g) the bath water being too hot or hot water being put in first;

(h) an unprotected hot-water bottle, or a hot-water bottle being left in a cot or pram with a sleeping child.

*Poisoning* may be due to:

(a) *Gas poisoning* from leaks, faulty fittings, children playing with gas taps, sleeping in a room with low gas-fire and inadequate ventilation;

(b) *Medicinal poisoning* from children eating tablets in mistake for sweets (especially ferrous sulphate, antihistamines, strychnine—in aperient and tonic pills—aspirin, barbiturates); taking medicines from unlabelled bottles or in the dark;

(c) *Household poisoning:* drinking by mistake cleaning materials or gardening preparations, especially if they have been put into soft-drink or other bottles and left within the reach of children; using any stain- or spot-remover containing carbon tetrachloride, which is in many of them, in an unventilated room, when smoking (the fumes can turn into phosgene), or before, during or after drinking any alcoholic drink (alcohol increases the absorption of carbon tetrachloride).

*Suffocation* (the commonest cause of accidental death in babies) may be due to:

(a) too large or too soft a pillow;

(b) overlaying by an adult who is sleeping in the same bed;

(c) not tucking in the bedclothes or tucking them in too tightly;

(d) inhalation of milk when a baby is left with a bottle propped in its mouth;

(e) putting a child to rest too soon after a feed and before it has brought up the wind, and putting the child on its back so that it is choked by any milk it brings up;

(f) plastic feeder sticking firmly over the baby's mouth;

(g) smothering by a cat lying on top of a baby.

*Electrical accidents* may be due to amateur installations and repairs, faulty plugs and flex, unearthed plugs, touching electrical equipment with wet hands, having electrical equipment in a bathroom, filling electric kettles without disconnecting them.

*Fireworks* are a common cause of injury. In England and Wales in 1974 over 800 people were injured by fireworks; although none died, nearly half sustained eye injuries. More than half the cases were children, a large proportion were injured at family or private parties and an equal number in casual incidents in the street. The eyes, the face and the hands were the parts most commonly burnt. Common causes of accidents were holding the firework in the hand, examining a firework to find out why it had not gone off, and the firework going off in a pocket. Greater care in handling and lighting fireworks and supervising children would have prevented many of these accidents.

*Gunshot accidents* are due to keeping guns loaded, careless handling, fooling about, pointing guns at people, and having faulty fire-arms.

## Prevention of Accidents

### General Principles

(a) Consider the home, every room in it, the ward and its annexes as possible sources of danger. Check all danger places. Have repairs carried out and extra lights put in dark places.

(b) Exercise proper supervision over small children and arrange help for the old and the physically handicapped.

(c) Have all electrical and gas fittings serviced by experts.

## Falls

1. Do not have slippery floors and loose mats.

2. Mend holes in carpets and linoleum.

3. Have adequate lighting with accessible switches.

4. Do not stand on rickety steps or chairs.

5. Do not allow things to lie on the floor where old people might trip over them.

6. Do not have trailing flexes.

7. Have rails attached to the sides of a bath for an old person to pull himself up with; have a rubber mat in the bath to prevent slipping on getting in and out.

8. See that stairs are kept in good repair and that carpet-rods are in place.

9. Wipe grease off the kitchen floor.

## Burns

1. Fit an adequate fireguard in front of electric fires, gas fires, coal fires and oil fires. Under the Heating Appliances (Fireguards) Act, 1952, it is illegal to sell electric, gas and oil fires without an approved guard, but fires bought before that Act came into force may not have an adequate guard.

2. See that an open coal fire has, where there are children or old people, a properly fitted guard that is fastened to the fireplace and cannot be moved away by a child. It is an offence to leave a child under 12 years of age in a room with an unguarded fire, although a prosecution can be made only if the child is burned.

3. Do not let children stay with friends or relatives who have unguarded fires.

4. Remember the fireguard when children are brought downstairs to sit by the fire when they have been ill or had a nightmare.

5. Do not dress or undress children in front of a fire.

6. Do not dress children in highly inflammable materials. Wear pyjamas rather than a nightie. Buy fire-resistant pyjamas or nighties for children.

7. Do not have a mirror over the mantelpiece in which a woman might be tempted to admire herself and in doing so set her dress on fire.

8. Do not leave matches lying about.

9. Do not leave an oil-stove in a draught or where it is likely to be knocked over.

10. Switch off an electric blanket before getting into bed and do not switch it on while in bed, unless it is of a type that can be left on all night.

### Scalds

1. Do not leave a child alone with a pot or cup of hot tea.

2. Do not have table-cloths for children; have mats or a plastic top to the table.

3. Have cooker and sink on the same side of the kitchen.

4. Do not pass hot liquids over anybody.

5. Do not let the flex of an electric kettle trail within reach of a crawler or toddler.

6. Buy saucepans with short grips on both sides rather than a long handle on one.

7. Keep saucepan handles and kettle spouts pointed inwards on stoves.

8. Fit on to the stove a metal guard, which can be pulled down to enclose the pans and so prevent children reaching them.

### Suffocation

1. Do not allow babies to have a pillow until they are about six months old and able to lift their heads off it. Do not let babies have plastic-covered mattresses or pillows.

2. Do not tuck them in too tightly or too loosely.

3. Never leave them alone with a bottle in the mouth.

4. Let them bring up wind after a meal and then lay them on their side.

5. Do not let them sleep in a bed with adults.

6. If there are cats about, get a net to stretch tightly over the pram.

7. Do not let children play with plastic bags which they might put over their heads and so suffocate themselves.

**Poisoning**

1. Keep all medicines in a locked cupboard high up or in an approved 'child-proof' poison cabinet.

2. Go through the cupboard and turn out unwanted or un-named tablets and medicines.

3. Warn children against eating tablets that look like sweets.

4. Check any medicine given.

5. Do not give or take any medicine or tablet whose nature you are not sure of.

6. Put tablets in boxes with spring-caps that children cannot easily open.

7. Do not put cleaning materials or garden liquids into soft-drink bottles.

8. Use a cleaner containing carbon tetrachloride only with doors and windows open, or preferably in the open air; do not smoke when using it; do not drink alcohol before, during or just after using it. Keep these cleaners away from children: a teaspoonful can be fatal to a small child.

# Chapter Thirteen

# THE PREVENTION OF INFECTION

Communicable diseases are specific diseases caused by micro-organisms and passed from one person to another either directly or by means of an intermediate agent; or communicated to man through other animals or from one animal to another. They may be spread by direct infection from man to man or indirectly by means of dust, milk, food, water, infected crockery, bedding, clothes and soil.

In all infections three factors have to be considered:

1. The source from which the infection arises.

2. The method of spread from one person to another.

3. The person who is infected.

Everybody exposed to an infection does not automatically develop the disease, and the disease itself may vary very much in the intensity with which it affects different people. At different times diseases may vary in their effects; scarlet fever, for example, which was formerly a serious infection with serious complications, has in recent years become comparatively mild. The *virulence* of the organism (that is, its ability to produce severe symptoms) depends on (a) the state of the organism itself, and (b) the ability of an infected person to stand up to it, which is called his *resistance*.

If a person is exposed to infection and gets the disease, he is said to have been *susceptible* to it; if he does not get it, he is regarded as being *immune* to it.

*Immunity* to an infection may be due to:

(a) *Natural Causes:*

1. A racial resistance to the disease, inherited from one's ancestors.

2. A previous attack of the disease.

3. Previous good health and nutrition.

(b) *An Artificial Cause:*

1. Having previously been given an inoculation to prevent the development of the disease.

A *carrier* is a person who carries on or in his body a harmful organism without being affected by it. This carrier-state may be temporary (as after an attack of cerebrospinal meningitis, when the organisms may linger in a virulent form in the throat for a short time) or permanent (as after an attack of typhoid fever, the organisms may live in the intestine and make the faeces infectious). Carriers are often the cause of fresh outbreaks of an infection.

The *incubation period* of an infectious disease is the period that elapses between the infection of a person and the appearance of the first symptoms. *Quarantine* is the period during which people who have been exposed to infection may be kept away from other people; it is usually the maximum incubation period plus two or three days.

A disease is said to be *sporadic* when single cases occur without any spread of the infection. It is *endemic* in an area or country when cases of it are continually occurring. It is *epidemic* when many cases occur in one place at one time and the disease spreads to other places. It is *pandemic* when it spreads all over the world.

### Notification of Communicable Diseases

The more serious of the communicable diseases are notifiable to the local Community Physician by the doctor who diagnoses them. The ones notifiable today in Britain are:

| | |
|---|---|
| Smallpox | Polio-encephalitis |
| Tuberculosis in any form | Cerebrospinal Meningitis |
| Typhoid and Paratyphoid | Scarlet Fever |
| Fevers | Diphtheria |
| Dysentery | Measles |
| Food Poisoning | Whooping Cough |
| Acute Primary | Erysipelas |
| Pneumonia | Ophthalmia Neonatorum |
| Influenzal Pneumonia | Infective Hepatitis |
| Acute Poliomyelitis | |

Some diseases rare here: Malaria, Relapsing Fever, Cholera, Plague, Encephalitis Lethargica, Typhus, Leprosy, Anthrax.

A number of very common communicable diseases are not notifiable because they are not usually serious, e.g. the common cold, German measles, mumps, impetigo, influenza (which is notifiable when it produces pneumonia), and chickenpox (except during epidemics of smallpox, when it may temporarily be made notifiable because a mild attack of smallpox is sometimes mistaken for chickenpox). Syphilis and gonorrhoea, although serious communicable diseases, are not notifiable.

## The Main Methods of Transmission

(a) *Air-borne*, e.g. pulmonary tuberculosis, smallpox, diphtheria, scarlet fever, whooping cough, mumps, chickenpox, influenza, the common cold. These diseases are spread mainly by the coughing, shouting, sneezing and laughter of an infected person. The organisms are sprayed out in tiny droplets of moisture (hence the term *droplet infection*) which another person may breathe in, or in smaller droplets which dry up, leaving an infectious dust on clothes, bedding, furnishings, crockery and floors.

(b) *By Food, Milk and Water*

*Food:* e.g. typhoid fever, paratyphoid fever, dysentery, staphylococcal food infections.

*Milk:* e.g. bovine tuberculosis, typhoid fever, paratyphoid fever, scarlet fever.

*Water:* e.g. typhoid fever, paratyphoid fever.

(c) *By Direct Contact:* e.g. impetigo (by kissing or embracing), syphilis and gonorrhoea (usually by sexual intercourse).

## The Control of Epidemics

A Community Physician becomes aware of an epidemic in his area by the notifications he receives, and he takes such measures as he can to prevent any further spread of it. He has three lines of attack:

to discover the source of the infection, to discover how it is spreading, and to protect the people exposed to infection.

*The Source.* The kind of notification he receives is often a clue to the source. For example, an epidemic of typhoid fever affecting children predominantly suggests a milk infection because children drink more milk than adults; and an epidemic of the same disease affecting men, women and children alike, especially if it is an explosive epidemic with many cases occurring simultaneously, suggests a water-borne infection, Suspicions may be confirmed by detailed laboratory investigations.

*Tracing the Spread.* Some diseases may be spread by direct contacts of the original case. This is particularly so in smallpox, an epidemic of which may be traced to one infected person who has brought the disease to an area or country.

*Isolation and Quarantine.* Isolation of a person suffering from a communicable disease may be necessary in order to check the spread of infection, e.g. for smallpox, typhoid fever, paratyphoid fever, and diphtheria. The spread of whooping cough, measles, and scarlet fever is not usually reduced by the isolation of patients, who may, however, have to be admitted into an isolation hospital if facilities for looking after them at home are inadequate.

Quarantine may be used for children exposed to infection in the form of keeping them away from nursery or school. Adults are not usually put into quarantine. Family contacts of a case of typhoid or paratyphoid fever should not handle food or do any cooking.

*Disinfection.* Excreta, surgical dressings, clothing, any articles used by the patient, and the room he has been in may have to be disinfected.

*Inoculation.* Inoculation of contacts may be advisable, e.g. the vaccination of anyone who has been in contact with a case of smallpox.

## The Prevention of Infection by Inoculation

Inoculation (or vaccination) is the injection of a micro-organism into the body in order that an artificial immunity to the disease may be produced. When a person develops a communicable disease, he produces in his body *antibodies* against the organism that has caused the disease or against the toxic products of the organism. Antibodies are chemical substances, are 'specific' for each disease, and once formed may persist in the body for life. This is why some communicable diseases cannot be caught a second time. The organisms used in inoculations are either dead or weakened by laboratory methods to such an extent that they are incapable of producing the disease; but they are capable of stimulating the body to produce the appropriate antibodies, although not always as many as would be produced by an attack of the disease. In consequence if a person in whom this artificial immunity has been produced is exposed to that infection, either he does not develop the disease at all or he gets it in a very mild form.

Diseases against which inoculation is available are: smallpox, diphtheria, typhoid and paratyphoid fevers, whooping cough, measles, rubella, poliomyelitis, tuberculosis and tetanus.

Measles, smallpox, diphtheria, poliomyelitis, whooping cough, tuberculosis and tetanus are particularly liable to affect children, and it is possible to inoculate children against them all. Combined inoculations against (a) diphtheria, whooping cough and tetanus or (b) diphtheria and tetanus can be used. The timing of these inoculations is designed to provide the maximum immunity against each disease, to keep as low as possible the number of injections given to a child, and to avoid harmful reactions or complications, such as provoking an attack of poliomyelitis (*see* table, pp. 117–18).

As an illustration of the effects of immunization against diphtheria (begun in this country in 1940), these figures may be considered:

|  | Number of Cases of Diphtheria in a Year | Deaths a Year |
|---|---|---|
| Between 1936 and 1940 | 55,312 | 2,700 |
| In 1973 | 2 | 0 |

Such an improvement can be maintained only by an enthusiastic continuation of the immunization programme.

Inoculation against typhoid and paratyphoid fevers is given to those especially exposed to risk, such as doctors and nurses in isolation hospitals, to troops and to people going to countries where the diseases are endemic.

## Cross Infection

The term 'cross infection' is used to describe the infection of a patient with a communicable disease while he is in hospital. Originally used to describe cases in isolation hospitals, where, for example, a patient admitted for diphtheria might develop scarlet fever, it has now been extended to the acquiring of an infection while in hospital for any reason. The wards in which it is most likely to occur are fever wards, children's wards, maternity wards, and ear, nose and throat wards.

More cubicles, barrier nursing and bed isolation have been introduced to reduce the incidence of cross infection. In barrier nursing all the articles used by a patient are kept apart and not used by other patients; and gowns are worn by doctors and nurses when attending the patient. In bed isolation the patient's feeding, toilet and sanitary utensils are sterilized after use and are allowed to be used by other patients.

### Methods of Reducing Cross Infection

1. The provision of smaller wards and more one-bed wards.

2. Barrier nursing and bed isolation.

3. Adequate ventilation of wards.

4. Beds to be spaced with at least 12 feet between the middles of the beds.

5. All members of the staff to be instructed in the principles of hygiene and to carry them out.

6. Nurses and orderlies to be immunized against communicable diseases.

7. Children are not to be admitted into a ward if the risk of being infected in it is great.

8. The preparing of children's feeds and the changing of nappies are never to be done by the same nurse.

9. Nurses and orderlies are not to come into the ward if they are ill.

10. Masks are to be worn by the staff as they attend to a patient with an air-borne infection.

11. No dressings are to be done until half an hour after bed-making and ward-cleaning so that dust can settle.

12. Bedclothes are kept off the floor.

13. Dusters are to be damped.

14. Soiled linen must not be counted or sorted in the ward.

15. Ward floors should be oiled with spindle oil, which keeps down the dust.

## Disinfection

Disinfection is the killing of harmful micro-organisms. Sterilization is the destruction of all micro-organisms. An antiseptic is a substance that prevents the growth of micro-organisms. A deodorant is a smell-remover. A detergent is a cleansing agent which cleanses by its special properties of wetting, emulsifying and dirt-suspending.

Disinfection can be carried out by boiling, burning, chemical methods, steam, dry heat and ultra-violet light.

**Boiling** for five minutes is used for most instruments, household utensils, feeding equipment, and for clothing, sheets and pillow-cases from which stains (such as blood-stains) that are liable to be 'fixed' by boiling have been removed.

**Burning** is used for soiled dressings, swabs soiled with excretions and secretions, paper handkerchiefs, and sputum cartons.

### Chemical Disinfection

*Phenol* (carbolic acid) is an antiseptic, disinfectant and deodorant. In dilutions of one in twenty it is used to disinfect bedpans, drains, surgical instruments and soiled linen. In strong concentrations it is irritant and caustic.

*Cresol* is used for the same purposes as Phenol, usually in the forms of Lysol (diluted one in a hundred) or Izal (diluted one in two hundred).

*Dettol* (used in dilutions of one in a hundred) is a synthetic antiseptic of the chloroxylene group. It is more powerful than the cresol group and less irritating to tissues.

*Cetrimide* (trade name: Cetavlon) is an antiseptic, a detergent and a deodorant. In strengths normally used it is colourless, odourless and tasteless: it is neither irritating nor toxic. In a dilution of one in a hundred it is used for cleaning the skin before an operation.

*Chlorine* is a strong antiseptic, disinfectant and deodorant. In the form of chlorinated lime (bleaching powder) it is used to disinfect water, swimming-pools, drains and privies. Chlorine gas is used to disinfect water-supplies. Eusol, Milton and Parazone are hypochlorite compounds that are disinfectants and deodorants.

*Formaldehyde* (formalin) is used as a vapour to sterilize rooms.

**Steam** is used to sterilize surgical dressings and to disinfect mattresses, pillows, blankets, clothing and other textiles. An *autoclave* is the apparatus in which this is done. It consists of an inner chamber into which the articles to be sterilized or disinfected are put and an outer chamber called the jacket. Steam at 20–30 lb. pressure per square inch and at 250° F (121° C) is introduced first into the jacket to heat the inner surface of the chamber and prevent condensation; a vacuum is then produced in the inner chamber, and steam is passed into it and kept in it at a pressure of 20–30 lb. per square inch and a temperature of 250° F (121° C) for twenty minutes. The articles in the *autoclave* are then dried by hot air, after which they can be taken out.

**Hot Air** sterilization, using a hot-air oven for 1 hour at 160° C., is the best method of sterilizing glassware of all kinds, and is particularly useful for all glass syringes. It can also be used for needles, scalpels, scalpel blades, scissors, forceps and other surgical instruments. It cannot be used for plastic materials, some nylon syringes, rubber materials and gum catheters, which cannot resist the heat reached in the oven. Petroleum jelly gauze may be sterilized by $2\frac{1}{2}$ hours in the oven.

**Ultra-Violet Light** is used to sterilize the air in wards where sterility is especially necessary, e.g. wards for premature babies.

## Disinfection of Articles

1. Scraps of food should be burnt.

2. Dressings, swabs from nose, throat and ear, sanitary towels, paper handkerchiefs and sputum cartons should be burnt.

3. Sputum in metal pots should be mixed with phenol solution, diluted one in twenty, for two hours and then poured down a drain. If a sputum-sterilizing *autoclave* is available, the sputum pot with its contents should be exposed to a pressure of 20 lb. per square inch at a temperature of 250° F (121° C) for twenty minutes.

4. Faeces should be (a) mixed with an equal amount of phenol one in twenty, broken up with a stick, and allowed to stand for two hours before disposal down a drain; or (b) covered with bleaching powder, have water added, be broken up, and allowed to stand for two hours before burial in the ground; or (c) sterilized by steam in a steam sterilizer.

5. Urine should be mixed with phenol one in twenty and allowed to stand for two hours.

6. Feeding and other domestic utensils should be boiled for five minutes.

7. Mattresses, pillows and linen should be steam-disinfected. Blankets and other woollens should be soaked in phenol one in twenty or exposed to formalin vapour.

8. Rooms may be disinfected by thorough washing of the floor and paint with soap and water and then opening the windows to sun and air. In severe infections (such as smallpox) the Health Authority will disinfect the room by formalin vapour. This involves opening all cupboards and drawers, freely exposing all articles in the room, including blankets, toy and leather articles, liberating formalin vapour by the heating of Paraform tablets (thirty 1 gram tablets per thousand feet of space), and leaving the room sealed up for six hours.

## The Prevention of Specific Infections

### Bacillary Dysentery

*Cause:* the dysentery bacillus, of which the four main groups are:

   *Shigella sonnei:* causes most cases in England;

*Shigella flexneri:* causes about one third of cases in Scotland;

*Shigella dysenteriae* and *Shigella boydii:* occur mainly in tropical countries and occasionally imported into Britain.

*Spread by:* faecal infection from acute patients or carriers or from contaminated articles; in the tropics by food contaminated by flies.

*Incubation period:* 1–7 days. The patient is infectious during the incubation period as well as the acute stage of the disease.

*Prevention:* washing hands after defaecation; good sanitation; hygienic methods of food distribution and preparation; detection of carriers; destruction of flies.

## Chickenpox

*Cause:* a virus; the same virus causes herpes zoster in later life.

*Spread by:* droplet infection from the air-passages.

*Incubation period:* usually 15–18 days.

*Prevention:* the illness is mild and no special precautions are necessary.

## Common Cold

*Cause:* a virus.

*Spread by:* droplet infection from the air-passages.

*Incubation period:* 1–3 days.

*Prevention:* people with colds should go to bed or at least keep away from other people.

## Diphtheria

*Cause:* a bacillus, *Co. diphtheriae*, of which there are several types with varying degrees of virulence.

*Spread by:* droplet infection, contaminated articles, carriers.

*Incubation period:* 1–6 days.

*Prevention:* (a) FT (Formol Toxoid) given to children in combination with other vaccines (see Schedule of Immunizations, pp. 117–18); (b) TAF (Toxoid-Antitoxin Floccules) in 3 doses of 1 ml, 1 ml, and 1·5 ml, with 3–4 weeks between injections; used for adults as it is less likely to produce unpleasant reactions in them.

**Erysipelas**

*Cause:* a streptococcus.

*Spread by:* direct contact.

*Incubation period:* 1–7 days.

*Prevention:* cleanliness of the skin; not scratching; avoidance of overcrowding.

**Food Poisoning**

*Causes:* Salmonella bacilli (named after a microbiologist, not after tinned salmon); and staphylococci.

*Spread by:* (a) Salmonella infections by man, dogs, cats, cattle, pigs, poultry, rats, duck eggs, pet foods, garden fertilizers; (b) staphylococcal infections by food (usually cold meat, milk, custard, ice cream) infected from the hands, face, nose or throat of someone preparing or handling it.

*Incubation periods:* Salmonella 12–24 hours; staphylococcus 1–6 hours.

*Prevention:* cleanliness in the preparation of food; washing the hands after defaecation; washing the hands after using garden fertilizer; no handling of food or cooking by a person with a staphylococcal infection; keeping raw pet food away from food intended for human consumption.

**German Measles [Rubella]**

*Cause:* a virus.

*Spread by:* droplet infection.

*Incubation period:* 12–18 days.

*Prevention:* vaccination of all girls at 11–14 years (whether they are thought to have had German measles or not) to prevent the transmission to any child they might bear, as the child of a woman who develops German measles during the early months of pregnancy has a 1 in 10 chance of being mentally retarded or having a physical defect such as congenital heart disease or deafness.

**Gonorrhoea**

*Cause:* the gonococcus.

*Spread by:* sexual intercourse; young girls are occasionally infected accidentally e.g. from a towel; a baby's eyes may be infected as it is being born.

*Incubation period:* 2–10 days.

*Prevention:* abstention of infected person from sexual intercourse; wearing of a sheath by the male; prompt treatment of infected persons; tracing and investigation of sexual partners of an infected person.

### Influenza

*Cause:* a virus, of which there are 3 main types: type A (the commonest), type B, type C.

*Spread by:* droplet infection from the air-passages.

*Incubation period:* 1–2 days.

*Prevention:* by vaccination, but the vaccine has to be of the appropriate strain.

### Measles

*Cause:* a virus.

*Spread by:* droplet infection from the air-passages.

*Incubation period:* about 11 days.

*Prevention:* a vaccine is given to children at 2 years if they have not had measles. Temporary immunity is provided for young children in poor health who have been exposed to infection by giving immunoglobulin intramuscularly.

### Meningococcal Meningitis Cerebrospinal Meningitis

*Cause:* the meningococcus.

*Spread by:* droplet infection, often from a carrier.

*Incubation period:* 1–3 days.

*Prevention:* adequate ventilation of schools, camps and barracks; isolation of patient; isolation of any contact until his naso-pharynx has been found not to contain meningococci; treatment of carriers.

### Mumps

*Cause:* a virus.

*Spread by:* droplet infection.

*Incubation period:* 14–21 days.

*Prevention:* patients should be isolated until 3 days after the parotid gland swelling has subsided.

## Poliomyelitis

*Cause:* a virus.

*Spread by:* direct contact; faecal infection of food and water; flies and cockroaches.

*Incubation period:* 7–12 days.

*Prevention:* vaccination with an oral vaccine of the Sabin type of virus with 3 doses of 3 drops each at intervals of 4–8 weeks. No other immunizing procedure is performed within 3 weeks and 'cold' (non-urgent) surgery is not carried out during the course.

## Scarlet Fever

*Cause:* streptococcus.

*Spread by:* droplet infection; discharge from ear, nose or throat; milk.

*Incubation period:* usually 2–4 days.

*Prevention:* isolation of patient at home for about 1 week.

## Serum Hepatitis

*Cause:* an unidentified virus referred to as virus B.

*Spread by:* blood of people carrying the virus, potentially infectious people are identified by being Australian antigen positive.

*Incubation period:* 40–150 days.

*Prevention:* identification of people who are Australian antigen positive; special precautions so that their blood does not come into contact with the blood of anyone else; special precautions in hospital with people of those groups known to have a high incidence of Australian antigen positive; the use of disposable syringes and needles; safe disposal of needles and other 'sharps' (any sharp instrument) after use so that no-one is pricked by them; the washing of blood off the hands immediately if any gets on them from anyone else; immediate reporting for investigation and treatment of any member of staff who pricks or cuts himself.

### Smallpox [Variola]

*Cause:* a virus, of which there are two main types: variola major virus which causes a severe and often fatal illness, and variola minor virus, which causes a milder illness.

*Spread by:* skin of patient, dust and clothing.

*Incubation period:* 11–14 days.

*Prevention:* (a) vaccination is recommended for people likely to come into contact with smallpox or living in or travelling to countries where it occurs; immunity lasts for 3–5 years; the international certificate of vaccination is valid for 3 years; (b) isolation of patient in an isolation hospital; disinfection of his room and clothing; (c) tracing and vaccination of contacts.

### Syphilis

*Cause:* a spirochete.

*Spread by:* sexual intercourse; occasionally by accidental contact.

*Incubation period:* 2–4 weeks.

*Prevention:* abstention of infected persons from sexual intercourse; prompt treatment; tracing and investigation of sexual partners of infected persons.

### Tetanus [Lockjaw]

*Cause:* a bacillus.

*Spread by:* infection of wounds by contaminated soil; occasionally by infection of surgical wounds at operation.

*Incubation period:* usually 2–28 days, can be longer.

*Prevention:* (a) Active immunization with tetanus toxoid in three injections of 1 ml each at intervals of 6 to 12 weeks and 6 to 12 months respectively between doses for people at risk—farm and garden workers, soldiers; subsequently a booster dose of 1 ml every 2 years. For children see Schedule of Immunizations, pp. 117–18; (b) passive immunization by an intramuscular injection of tetanus antitoxin 1500–3000 international units to non-immunized people who have received a wound likely to be contaminated with soil. The patient's sensitivity to the antitoxin is tested before immunization.

**Typhoid Fever**

*Cause:* a bacillus.

*Spread by:* faecal contamination of water or food; bedpans, enema syringes, bedding; laboratory workers by their own cultures.

*Incubation period:* 10–12 days.

*Prevention:* (a) The provision of a safe water supply; pasteurization of milk; handwashing after defaecation and before the preparation of food or eating; the sanitary disposal of human excreta; the extermination of flies. (b) The isolation of the patient; the detection of carriers; the prevention of carriers from having anything to do with food. (c) Immunization by 2 injections of 0·5 ml vaccine of those exposed to infection, followed by booster doses every 3 years.

(Vaccination against paratyphoid fever, a similar but milder disease, is not very effective, causes unpleasant reactions, and is not recommended.)

**Whooping Cough [Pertussis]**

*Cause:* a bacillus.

*Spread by:* droplet infection.

*Incubation period:* 7–14 days.

*Prevention:* by immunization in infancy; see Schedule of Immunizations, below.

## Schedule of Immunizations

Vaccines are available for the immunization of children against diphtheria, measles, whooping cough, tetanus, smallpox, poliomyelitis, tuberculosis.

In order to reduce the number of injections necessary while providing maximum benefit for as many children as possible, it is usual to combine some of the injections. The following is one scheme.

| Age | Vaccine | Number |
|---|---|---|
| 3 to 6 months | (a) combined diphtheria, tetanus, whooping cough; (b) oral poliomyelitis | 3 at intervals of 4 to 8 weeks |

| Age | Vaccine | Number |
|---|---|---|
| 1 to 2 years | (a) & (b) booster doses; (c) measles | 1 of each |
| 5 years | (a) & (b) booster doses | 1 of each |
| 8 to 12 years | (a) & (b) booster doses | 1 of each |
| 12 years (earlier if exposed to infection | BCG for children who are tuberculin-negative | 1 only |
| 11 to 14 years (girls) | German measles | 1 only |

# Chapter Fourteen

# TUBERCULOSIS

Tuberculosis is an infectious disease of especial importance, one of the scourges of man, and probably responsible for one death in eight throughout the world. It is due to infection with the Bacillus tuberculosis, of which two different types affect man:

1. The *human type*, which is the chief cause of pulmonary tuberculosis;

2. The *bovine type*, which is the chief cause of tubercular adenitis, especially of the abdomen.

Other types of the tuberculosis bacillus affect birds, voles and other animals, but do not affect man.

**The human type** causes tuberculosis in man, monkeys, pigs and occasionally dogs and parrots. It is responsible for about 90 per cent of all cases of pulmonary tuberculosis and about 75 per cent of cases of non-pulmonary tuberculosis. Infection is spread by the sputum of people suffering from pulmonary tuberculosis, either directly from person to person by coughing, sneezing, shouting or laughing or indirectly by infected dust, the result of the drying of tiny droplets. The bacilli are quickly killed by sunlight and ordinary washing processes, but they can persist for months on the outer clothing, bedspread, curtain and rugs on which droplets of infected sputum have fallen. They persist longest in dark and damp places.

**The bovine type** occurs in man, cattle, pigs and horses. It is responsible for 60 to 70 per cent of all cases of tubercular adenitis (infection of the lymphatic glands) and for 10 to 20 per cent of all cases of bone and genito-urinary tuberculosis. Bovine infection is spread by the drinking of infected, untreated milk from tuberculous cows. Cows are particularly liable to spread the infection if they have tuberculous udders. Tuberculosis of cows can be a common infection in those countries where there are inadequate measures to control it (see p. 33). In some countries (e.g. Britain and the U.S.A.) the disease has been practically eradicated.

The social conditions associated with a high incidence of tuberculosis are overcrowding, poverty and malnutrition; and improvements in standards of living are usually followed by a reduction in the number of cases. In countries where social and working conditions are good and people are well fed, the incidence of the disease has been on the decline for many years, with the exception of the years during and immediately after the world wars when the incidence increased due to a deterioration in social conditions, overcrowding, loss of houses, and a diminution in the amount of food available. In Britain the incidence of the disease is falling, and during the last thirty years the number of deaths from it has fallen sharply, probably as a result of such factors as: (a) the discovery of early or symptomless cases by mass radiography; (b) immunization by B.C.G. vaccine; (c) new methods of chemotherapy using combinations of three drugs, streptomycin, para-amino-salicylic acid (PAS) and iso-nicotinic acid; (d) better social conditions, and (e) the eradication of bovine tuberculosis.

However, mass radiography findings suggest that there are in Britain today several thousand cases of unrecognized active tuberculosis in persons over the age of fifteen, of whom a little more than a third might be infectious. Moreover, immigrants from countries such as Pakistan, where tuberculosis is common, may be infected before they come to this country, bring the infection with them, and be liable to infect other people with whom they associate. In 1973 the number of notified cases in England and Wales was 10,576, but the number of deaths from tuberculosis (1,240) was the lowest ever recorded.

Infants have little or no natural resistance to tuberculosis, but start to develop some resistance several months after birth. With the diminution of infection by bovine tuberculosis, children are not so liable to develop the disease as are adolescents, especially girls; and there is now in this country a high incidence of the disease in men over forty.

The incidence of the disease in industrialized communities ensured that most people came into contact with it during their early life and developed a childhood primary complex of a nodule (the typical 'tubercle' from which the disease gets its name) in a lung and involvement of the lymph glands at the root of the lung. Most of these infections do not produce any symptoms, the person does not know he has been infected, and the tuberculous lesions heal. Enough 'resistance' may have been developed in the person's tissues to ensure that he does not again succumb to the infection, but he will be otherwise still liable to develop the much more severe, dangerous and infectious pulmonary tuberculosis of the adult if his resistance is not strong enough to withstand fresh infection either from another person or from the quiescent primary infection in his lung reawakening into activity. In primitive communities, where the people have not previously been exposed to infection and been able to build up resistance to it, tuberculosis is likely to spread at first in epidemic form as an acute disease with a high mortality and then, some time later, to assume the more chronic form. In impoverished countries and the tropics tuberculosis affects many million people in an active form. The methods by which its incidence can be reduced are:

(a) an improvement in economic and social conditions;

(b) a knowledge of the nature of the disease and the measures that will prevent infection;

(c) the early diagnosis of cases;

(d) modern methods of chemotherapeutic treatment.

### Diagnosis

The diagnosis is usually made on clinical grounds and the evidence of X-rays and blood tests. A definite diagnosis can be made by the discovery of the tubercle bacillus in the sputum, on a laryngeal swab, or in the stomach wash-outs and faeces of children and mental patients that swallow their sputum.

**Tuberculin Tests** on the skin are used to determine a patient's sensitivity to tuberculin, as an indication of previous infection and the acquirement of immunity. The tests are based upon the fact that infection by tuberculosis makes the tissues of the body super-sensitive to the toxins of the bacillus with a sensitivity that persists for life. Tuberculin is obtained from the fluid in which tubercle bacilli have been grown in a laboratory; it does not contain tubercle bacilli. The recommended form of tuberculin is Purified Protein Derivative (PPD). The test may be done in several ways.

In the *Heaf Test* an automatic punch is used which has six needles set in a small circle. For children under two years of age the needles can be set to penetrate 1 mm into the skin, and for older people they can be set to penetrate 2 mm. To perform the test, a small area of skin on the forearm or thigh is cleansed with spirit or acetone. A sterile platinum loop or glass rod is used to transfer a little PPD on to the skin and to spread it in a film over a circular area about 1 cm in diameter. The punch is set to puncture to the required depth, the disc is placed over the film and held firmly on, and the handle is pressed. The needles are thus driven into the skin; the operation is painless. The film is allowed to dry, no dressing being required. The reaction can be read at any time between 72 hours and 7 days. A positive reaction is shown by the occurrence of induration, which can be felt with the tip of a finger, over at least four of the six puncture marks; if the test has been properly performed all six points will be indurated. Absence of induration over four points is a negative reaction.

In the *Tine Test* a plastic applicator on whose four needlepoints tuberculin has been allowed to dry is pressed on to the skin by hand; the applicator is used only once.

The *Mantoux Test* is another tuberculin test. In this test 0·1 ml of 1/10,000 of PPD is injected with a tuberculin syringe and an intradermal needle into the skin of the forearm. The site of the injection is inspected 72 hours later (in a few people the reaction may not appear for another 24 hours). A positive reaction is one in which a raised area of induration not less than 6 mm in diameter appears. The raised area is surrounded by a zone of erythema; erythema alone is not a positive reaction. If the test is negative, the test is repeated with PPD 1/1,000 dilution. If this second injection is negative, it can be assumed that the person has not had tuberculosis and has not acquired any immunity to the disease.

## The Prevention of Tuberculosis

1. *Better Housing.* As tuberculosis is associated with overcrowding, houses or flats should be built with an adequate number of bedrooms. Preferably not more than two people and certainly not more than three should have to sleep in one room.

2. *Good Nutrition.* Well-fed people of good nutrition do not develop tuberculosis as easily as the thin or the half-starved. An inadequate diet is usually the result of poverty and ignorance of nutritional requirements and food values.

3. *The Early Diagnosis of Infection.* Mass Radiography is the most important single method of diagnosing early infection of the lungs. Mass Radiography Units are designed to take X-rays of the chest on miniature film at the rate of up to a hundred people an hour. If an abnormality is found on the miniature film, a full size X-ray is subsequently taken.

4. *The provision of Safe Milk.* Milk can be made safe to drink if it is pasteurized or sterilized, by which processes any tubercle bacilli present will be killed. The eradication of tuberculosis in cows will prevent infection of milk at the source, but because of the liability of cows to develop the disease heat treatment of milk is the only safe way of ensuring its freedom from tubercle bacilli.

5. *Ventilation in Industry.* Tuberculosis may be a complication of the pneumoconioses or dust diseases. The incidence of these diseases can be reduced by improvements in ventilation and techniques designed to prevent the inhalation of dangerous dusts (see Chapter 17).

6. *Tuberculin Testing* of children, nurses, other hospital staff, and people especially likely to develop tuberculosis, e.g. sailors.

7. *Immunization of Negative-Tuberculin Reactors.* People who do not show a positive reaction to the Tuberculin Test are particularly liable to be seriously infected by the first infectious case of tuberculosis they come into contact with and should be immunized against tuberculosis. This can be done by the use of a vaccine:

*The Bacillus Calmette-Guérin Vaccine* (BCG) is the one usually used. This vaccine is a bovine strain of the bacillus whose virulence has been weakened by cultivation in adverse conditions. The dose is 0·1 ml given intradermally. BCG is issued only to chest physicians, paediatricians, medical officers in charge of hospital staff, and community physicians. In tropical countries a freeze-dried BCG vaccine may be used or a heat-resistant or isoniazid-resistant BCG vaccine, the latter being used with oral isoniazid for breast-fed infants who are contacts with a known case of tuberculosis.

A satisfactory injection produces a small weal. No dressing is required. A small papule develops at the site and may ulcerate and then require a dressing.

Immunization in this way causes most tuberculin-negative people to become tuberculin-positive in about six weeks, a change that is believed to indicate a development of resistance to tuberculosis.

### Provisions for Treatment

The Area Health Authority, acting through the Community Physician and his staff, is responsible for prevention and after-care. Cases of tuberculosis are notified to the Community Physician. His Health Visitor visits the home of a notified case, advises the parents and relatives on the precautions they should take, reports on the housing and sleeping conditions, follows up contacts, and arranges for them to be X-rayed. After a patient's discharge from hospital or sanatorium the Health Visitor periodically visits him at home and offers advice about further care and precautions.

Assistance can be given in obtaining suitable housing accommodation; the children of infected parents can be boarded out; extra food, clothing and bedding can be provided for necessitous families; and patients are put into touch with the local Disablement Resettlement Officer, who will try to arrange suitable employment, and other services.

**Drug Treatment.** It is very important that a patient should know that if he continues to take drugs as prescribed he will almost certainly be cured. But courses of treatment last a long time and it is difficult to persuade some people to take tablets or cachets when they are feeling perfectly well, and there are many defaulters from treatment.

The usual method of treatment is to give:

(a) for the first 2–3 months a combination of three drugs: streptomycin by injection and isoniazid and PAS by mouth;

(b) for the next 18–24 months a combination of two drugs, usually isoniazid and PAS.

Drug resistance rarely develops when two or three drugs are taken together. Other drugs (e.g. thiacetazone) can be given if resistance should develop to any of the others.

Chapter Fifteen

# ALCOHOL, TOBACCO, DRUGS

Alcohol, tobacco, and drugs taken for non-medical reasons are threats to health.

## Alcohol

The alcohol in alcoholic drinks is ethyl alcohol. Alcoholic drinks are made by (a) the fermentation of cereals or fruits, (b) by distillation, (c) by mixing wine with brandy, etc. to produce fortified wine such as port.

The amount of alcohol in drink is:

| | |
|---|---|
| beer | 4–6 per cent |
| wine | 10–12 per cent |
| spirits (whisky, gin, brandy, etc) | 40–45 per cent |
| fortified wine | 15–22 per cent |

**Alcohol in the Body.** Alcohol is absorbed from the stomach and small intestine. The rate of absorption is rapid, but it is affected by the presence of food in the stomach, by the rate of gastric emptying, and by the amount and type of drink taken. Alcohol is transported by the portal system of veins to the liver and thence into the rest of the body in the general circulation. It is eventually oxidized in the liver into carbon dioxide and water. The larger the liver the more rapidly does oxidation take place. Taking fructose, found, for example, in fruits and honey, is the only known way to increase the rate of oxidation. About 5 per cent of alcohol drunk is eliminated as such, most of it by the kidneys. Alcohol can provide energy, but it has no other value as a food; it is not stored in the body.

There is a steady ratio between the amount of alcohol in the blood and the amount in the alveolar air, and breath tests for alcohol are used to determine the amount of alcohol in the blood. In

Britain it is illegal to drive a car with an alcohol level of 80 mg per 100 ml of blood or above.

## Physical Effects of Alcohol

*Stomach.* Small amounts of alcohol increase the secretion of gastric juice, hence the use of alcoholic drinks as appetizers. Large amounts cause gastritis and vomiting. Prolonged excessive drinking causes chronic gastritis, which interferes with the digestion of food.

*Heart and circulation.* Small amounts increase the heart rate and raise the blood pressure. Large amounts impair the circulation. Very large amounts can cause shock.

*Skin.* Dilatation of the blood vessels causes warmth and flushing.

*Nervous system.* All functioning of the nervous system is depressed.

*Liver.* Excessive drinking impairs liver function.

*Kidneys.* Urine production is increased while the blood alcohol is rising.

**Psychological Effects of Alcohol.** The psychological effects are related to the level of alcohol in the blood, e.g.:

| Alcohol per 100 ml blood | Effect |
| --- | --- |
| 20 mg | cheerfulness |
| 40 | driving ability at speed impaired |
| 50 | loss of inhibitions |
| 80 | deterioration of motor reactions |
| 100 | unsteadiness, lessened adaptation to darkness |
| 150 | obvious drunkenness |
| 300 | stupor |
| 500 | coma |

### Alcoholism

A person can be considered an alcoholic when his life is dominated by drinking and when he cannot control the amount he drinks and the number of times he drinks. Some alcoholics have bouts of heavy drinking followed by periods of abstinence, others are chronic tipplers who drink to excess all the time. Many alcoholics were originally unstable people, but stable people can become alcoholics especially if their work is by custom one in which drinking is common. People particularly likely to become alcoholics because of their work are: people in the liquor trade, sales representatives, senior executives in firms, journalists, and merchant navy seamen.

Women likely to become alcoholics are the wives of senior executives, women living alone, divorced women. The children of alcoholics are liable to become alcoholics because of being brought up in a home where drinking is common.

The incidence of alcoholism in a country is assessed from: deaths from alcoholism, admissions into hospital for alcoholism and alcoholic psychoses, deaths from cirrhosis of the liver (of which alcohol is the usual cause), and convictions for drunkenness and driving when drunk.

At a modest estimate there are 400,000 alcoholics in England and Wales and 75,000 in Scotland. The number is increasing. About 5 per cent of all alcoholics are socially grossly deteriorated, 'skid row' alcoholics.

**Clinical Features of Alcoholism.** Alcoholism causes psychological and behavioural abnormalities and physical abnormalities.

*Psychological and behavioural abnormalities* include:
    intellectual deterioration
    emotional disturbances, resentment, jealousy
    outbursts of rage and aggression
    delusions about spouse's fidelity
    threats of suicide
    frequent changes of employment
    Monday morning absenteeism
    frequent car accidents

*Physical abnormalities* include:

| flushed face | breath smelling of drink |
|---|---|
| nocturnal sweating | bruising and cigarette burns |
| blackouts | anaemia |

| | |
|---|---|
| obesity | degeneration of heart |
| vitamin deficiencies | peripheral neuropathy |
| pancreatitis | cirrhosis of liver |
| delirium tremens | dementia |

**Treatment of Alcoholism.** The treatment of alcoholism is difficult and many patients relapse. The essential features of treatment are:

(a) to persuade the patient that he is ill and that his illness is due to excessive drinking;

(b) to induce him to stop drinking and to be abstinent for life;

(c) to treat the 'abstinence syndrome' (anxiety, restlessness, tremor, sometimes fits) which lasts for a few days after stopping heavy drinking.

(d) if necessary to refer the patient to hospital for detoxication ('drying out') or for special treatment;

(e) to correct any anaemia or vitamin deficiency;

(f) to suggest to the patient that he gets into touch with Alcoholics Anonymous, a self-help organization of ex-alcoholics. Al-Anon is a similar organization to help the spouse of an alcoholic.


## Tobacco

Smoking is a serious danger to health. Cigarettes are the most dangerous form of tobacco. Smoking can cause:

*Cancer of the lung.* The incidence of deaths from cancer of the lung in England and Wales rose from 8,000 in 1946 to over 30,000 in 1973, of whom one-fifth were women, cancer of the lung being in them the second commonest cause of death from cancer (the first being cancer of the breast).

Smoking can also cause *cancer of the larynx*, and *cancer of the lip* in a pipe smoker.

Smoking is an important factor in the causation of: *chronic bronchitis* and *respiratory failure*; *angina pectoris* due to spasm of the coronary arteries of the heart; *thrombo-angiitis obliterans*, a disease in which the blood vessels of the legs become blocked; *failure of healing of a peptic ulcer.*

Smoking by a woman during pregnancy can damage the child

and cause: *retardation of growth, premature birth*, and *increased risk of perinatal death from any cause.* In England and Wales about 1,500 babies die every year because their mothers smoked during pregnancy.

*Passive smoking* is the inhalation of tobacco smoke puffed out by someone else. One cigarette can contaminate the air of a room, and smoking can be dangerous to the non-smoker. Particularly at risk are the babies of parents who smoke, and in them the incidence of respiratory illness is much higher than in the babies of non-smoking parents.

**Treatment.** Treatment is to stop smoking. This is done by an effort of will and a refusal to accept the blandishments of advertisers. Cigarettes with a low tar content may be less dangerous than those with a high tar content, and those who cannot give up smoking should switch to them.

### Drugs

The taking of drugs for non-medical reasons can be a cause of much ill-health, abnormal behaviour and premature death. Drugs commonly taken are:

| | |
|---|---|
| barbiturates | cannabis |
| lysergide (LSD) | amphetamine |
| heroin | cocaine |
| morphine | pethidine. |

An addict may take more than one drug at a time or switch from one drug to another as they become available, and he may take alcohol to excess as well as take drugs. Addicts who take drugs by injection are very likely to develop boils, sepsis, serum hepatitis and pneumonia, and to die young; there is a high incidence of Australian antigen positive in them.

The *Misuse of Drugs Act 1971* is the principal Act designed to control the use of addictive drugs and to prevent drug abuse.

**Barbiturates** are depressants of the brain and spinal cord. In small doses they impair higher nervous functions; in moderate doses they cause clouding of consciousness and sleep; in large doses they cause death by paralysing the cardiac and respiratory centres. They have usually been prescribed in the first place by a doctor for the relief of anxiety, depression or insomnia. The clinical features of barbiturate poisoning are similar to those of alcoholic intoxication, and many a person has killed himself by washing down his nightly dose of barbiturate with a stiff alcoholic drink.

**Cannabis** is the commonest drug used illicitly in Britain and it is usually smoked. People who smoke it do it to make themselves 'high', i.e. relaxed and euphoric. Taking it affects their ability to drive cars and control machinery. It is the drug of preference of students and middle-class bohemians who claim that it does them no harm, that it does not interfere with the attainment of social and intellectual aims, that it does not lead to taking other drugs, and that it is possible to give it up without too much difficulty. Little is known of its long-term effects.

**Lysergide** (LSD) is much more serious in its effects than cannabis. It is taken in very small doses and its effects last for 2–3 hours. These effects include: (a) a 'trip', which is characterized by altered consciousness, feelings of delight or terror, hallucinations and disturbed behaviour; a 'bad trip' is an attack of acute anxiety or terror; (b) intense chronic anxiety; (c) nausea, sweating, dizziness and changes in the pulse rate.

**Amphetamine** produces a state of wellbeing and self-confidence, and relieves fatigue; large amounts cause aggression and dangerous antisocial behaviour. Tolerance develops and to get the same effects a person has to take larger and larger amounts. Large doses produce restlessness, rapid speech, insomnia, tremor, rapid and irregular beating of the heart, paranoid ideas and hallucinations.

**Heroin** (diamorphine hydrochloride) produces a feeling of happiness and wellbeing. Addiction to it causes severe mental and physical deterioration.

**Cocaine** is usually taken alone or together with heroin. A 'sniff' of it produces a feeling of elation which lasts for about fifteen minutes and may be followed by a period of depression. It is expensive and in Britain taking it is limited to London and the 'pop world'.

**Morphine and pethidine.** Addiction to morphine and pethidine is not so common as addiction to the other drugs, but they may become the drugs of addiction of doctors, nurses and pharmacists who have access to them. Small doses produce a feeling of euphoria. Tolerance and mental and physical deterioration develop.

**Treatment** of drug addiction is very difficult and many patients relapse. Withdrawal from drugs can be carried out in hospital under supervision. Persuading the patient to abstain for the future, without the 'prop' of drugs, may require psychiatric techniques.

One of the claims of smokers of cannabis is that they can give it up without much trouble. Addicts to the 'hard' drugs are unlikely to give them up voluntarily for they are unwilling to endure the withdrawal symptoms and to give up a way of life in which drug-taking is a part.

# Chapter Sixteen

# PROVISIONS FOR THE DISABLED

Disablement is any impairment of capacity for life, work and enjoyment due to congenital defect, illness, or injury. It is difficult to assess the number of disabled persons in a community, but it is estimated that in Britain at least one person in ten and possibly as many as one in eight is disabled in one way or another.

Special provisions for disabled persons are provided in Britain by government departments, by professional organizations and voluntary societies. Among the government departments concerned are the Department of Health and Social Security, the Department of Employment, and the Department of Education and Science. The Department of Health is advised by a Committee on the Health and Welfare of Handicapped Persons and the Department of Employment by a National Advisory Council. Among the professional organizations concerned are the Queen's Nursing Institute, the Institute of Home Help Organisers, the Medical Society for the Care of the Elderly, the British Medical Association, and the Royal College of Psychiatrists. The many voluntary societies are concerned with the problems of disabled persons in general or of people with particular disabilities—the blind, deaf, mentally ill, mentally retarded, epileptics, spastics, autistic children, patients with muscular dystrophy, patients with multiple (disseminated) sclerosis, haemophiliacs, etc. The Central Council for the Disabled acts as a co-ordinating body of the various voluntary organizations, and the British Council for the Rehabilitation of the Disabled promotes the development of rehabilitation services by collecting and spreading information, by stimulating public action, and by holding conferences.

## Rehabilitation

Rehabilitation is the restoration of a person after illness or injury to full physical and mental function if it can be achieved.

Rehabilitary measures should be contemplated at the beginning of any disability and should include all measures that (a) minimize any loss of physical or mental function, (b) promote morale, (c) assist convalescent persons to regain full function and to resume their normal activities, and (d) help those left with a permanent disability to adjust to it and to live and work in conditions suited to their incapacity.

**Rehabilitation in Hospital.** The rehabilitation of a physically handicapped patient is usually directed by a specialist in physical medicine, who in consultation with the physician or surgeon in charge of the case works out a scheme of rehabilitation. The scheme is likely to include physiotherapy, remedial exercises, and possibly occupational therapy, all the activities being directed towards the patient's resuming if possible a normal life and going back to his old work or being trained for a new life and a new job. The rehabilitation of a psychiatric patient is directed by the consultant psychiatrist, and is likely to be by psychotherapy, occupational and industrial training, and training in social adaptation.

Case-conferences are held at which a patient's future and the measures to be taken to restore him if possible to active life are discussed by the doctor, a social worker, a physiotherapist, and when indicated, the Disablement Resettlement Officer from the local Job Centre. Attention is paid to the particular problems of the disabled housewife or the man who has to look after himself, especially the one-armed or chair-bound person. Training departments in hospital are fitted with training kitchens in which the furniture and utensils have been designed for use by a cripple; and in parts of the country special centres exist in which patients can be trained for work and normal activities and in overcoming the daily problems of dressing, washing, bathing, eating, travelling, running a home, and practising a hobby.

**Resettlement in Employment.** The Department of Employment has powers to help the disabled to obtain work and to provide industrial rehabilitation and vocational training. In each Job Centre a Register is kept of people who 'on account of injury, disease or congenital deformity' are 'substantially handicapped in obtaining or keeping employment' or of working on their own at a job which would be suitable for people of their age, ability and experience. At each Job Centre and Employment Rehabilitation Unit of the Department of Employment there is a Disablement Resettlement Officer (DRO) whose job is to advise disabled adults and help them to obtain suitable employment. People under 18 years of age are similarly advised by the Careers Officer. The DRO visits hospitals to advise handicapped persons who are about to be discharged, and he keeps in touch with local employers in order that he can be informed of any vacancy that a disabled person could fill. Employers of 20 or more persons must by law employ a quota of registered disabled persons. Certain kinds of employment (car park attendants, attendants on passenger electric lifts) are reserved for disabled persons. Most disabled persons if placed in suitable work can hold their own in competition with the able-bodied.

*Employment Rehabilitation Units* are now provided by the Employment Services Agency in several parts of the country. Their function is to condition and assess disabled persons for work in general, not for particular jobs. Each year over 10,000 persons enter these units for courses of rehabilitation which last usually for 7 to 8 weeks. The units are situated in places where there is the greatest need, and if the trainee cannot get to the unit, lodgings for him are provided and paid for; the person is paid while he is at the unit.

At such a unit the person has his physical condition assessed by a doctor, his abilities and aptitudes assessed by an industrial psychologist, his personal difficulties dealt with by a social worker.

The trainee's physical condition is improved by exercises in a gymnasium or by gardening, and his morale, which may have been shattered by his disability, is built up. At a weekly meeting chaired by the Rehabilitation Officer, the Unit Doctor, Occupational Psychologist, Disablement Resettlement Officer, Social Worker and Chief Occupational Supervisor discuss the results of their tests and interviews, and plan individual courses. At the end of the course they review progress and give a recommendation on future employment. This is sent in confidence to the Disablement Resettlement Officer (DRO) at the Job Centre so that local employers can be approached about suitable jobs. Sometimes the Employment Rehabilitation Unit (ERU) recommends training in a skilled grade, which is then arranged at a Government Skill Centre or elsewhere. The Employment Rehabilitation Unit does not undertake training.

Some large industrial firms (such as some car manufacturers) have rehabilitation units for their own employees.

A *Government Skill Centre* has different functions, including the training of suitable disabled persons in particular trades. The Centres are equipped with modern machinery, tools and equipment. Many of the Employment Rehabilitation Units are attached to Government Skill Centres, some of which have hostels. hostels.

Commercial and secretarial training can be arranged by the Department of Employment and is carried out in ordinary technical schools and secretarial colleges. For suitable candidates professional training, including studying for a university degree, can be arranged.

Among the voluntary organizations, the Royal National Institute for the Blind has a School of Physiotherapy in London and a college for training typists and telephonists. The Royal National Institute for the Deaf provides special homes and hostels, a training centre for maladjusted deaf youths, free testing of hearing-aids, and a special information service for the deaf. Other residential training centres in which various trades are taught to disabled persons are run by voluntary societies.

**Aids in the Home.** Many disabled persons have difficulties in the ordinary daily activities in the home. In its handbook *Practical Aids for the Disabled* the British Red Cross Society has provided information on making simple aids for disabled persons, many of them invented by disabled persons in order to overcome particular disabilities. In it details are given of aids for dressing (such as a long-handled comb, a long-handled lipstick, a stocking puller-on), aids for the bathroom (such as tap turner-on, a soap and sponge holder), in the kitchen (such as an aid for removing lids, a fruit and vegetable peeler), in the dining room (such as a padded spoon, an egg-stand for a boiled egg, a drinking aid) and for leisure hours (such as a writing board, a pencil-holder, a page-turner for spastics, a needle-stand). The devices are simple and could be easily made by a handy-man.

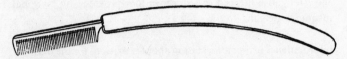

FIG. 23. *Long-handled comb. This aid is made from a wooden coat-hanger cut to the required length for the particular patient who needs it, with a tail comb inserted at one end, or attached to the hanger with screws*

The house in which a disabled person lives may have to be adapted, doors may have to be widened or ramps put over steps if the patient is in a wheelchair, the kitchen may have to be redesigned, a bathroom put on the ground-floor. Local Authorities have powers to carry out these alterations, to loan special equipment, and to provide home-nursing and domestic help.

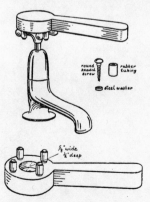

FIG. 24. *Tap-turner for a patient with a weak grip*

The *Chronically Sick and Disabled Persons Act 1970* directs that a Local Authority must inform itself of all chronically sick and disabled persons in its area and provide them with appropriate assistance such as meals, a telephone, wireless, television, library services, travelling facilities and holidays. Public buildings, universities and schools must be adapted or constructed so that disabled persons can use them, with entrances and lavatories for disabled persons and parking places for invalid cars.

**Financial Aid.** A disabled person may find his income sharply reduced. The ways in which financial aid is given are by (a) National Insurance Benefit, (b) Industrial Injuries Benefit, (c) War Pension, (d) payment while undergoing training in a Rehabilitation or Training Unit—such payment is higher than unemployment pay but less than normal pay for a job, and (e) Supplementary Allowances for those in need of aid above that provided by National Insurance Benefit.

**Information.** Further information about provisions for the disabled can be obtained from:

(a) The DRO or Careers Officer at any Job Centre;

(b) The British Red Cross Society, 9 Grosvenor Crescent, London, S.W.1;

(c) The Central Council for the Disabled, 34 Eccleston Square, London, S.W.1;

(d) The British Council for the Rehabilitation of the Disabled, Tavistock Square South, Tavistock Square, London, W.C.1.

# Chapter Seventeen

# INDUSTRIAL HYGIENE

Industrial hygiene is the application of the principles of hygiene to the health and welfare of workpeople and the protection of them from danger. Many branches of industry are associated with special risks and dangers, from inherent causes such as those of coal-mining, from the physical conditions under which work is done, and from chemical substances used in industry. Among the common causes and contributory factors of industrially produced ill health are: (a) poor factory conditions such as inadequate ventilation, inadequate lighting, faulty heating, noise and vibration; (b) fatigue and boredom; and (c) exposure to poisonous substances and the inhalation of toxic gases and dust.

## Industrial Medical Services

The Department of Employment is advised by the Health and Safety Commission; factories are inspected by medical and other specialist inspectors.

The publicly owned corporations and many private companies have their own industrial health services, staffed by doctors and nurses, and appropriate accommodation for carrying out medical examinations, treating casualties and doing minor operations. Smaller companies often employ a full-time nurse and a part-time medical officer, usually one of the local family doctors. Where no nurse is employed an industrial firm must have some responsible person trained in first aid.

Among the duties of an industrial medical officer are:

(a) The medical examination of employees under the age of eighteen, the medical examination of new entrants, and the medical examination of persons in known hazardous work.

(b) Arranging rehabilitation courses for workpeople who have been off work because of sickness or injury.

(c) The supervision of hygienic arrangements in the factory, with especial reference to known risks, cleanliness, lavatory accommodation, ventilation, heating, lighting, the provision of drinking water, the provision of washing facilities, and the wearing of protective clothing.

(d) The organization of adequate first-aid facilities.

(e) Advising management and workers on anything affecting health in the factory.

Several thousand nurses are employed in industry, many of them holding the Certificate in Occupational Health Nursing of the Royal College of Nursing or of the Birmingham Accident Hospital. The duties of a nurse in a factory include assisting the medical officer in his examinations, maintaining the ambulance rooms and casualty arrangements in a state of readiness, giving first-aid treatment, educating workpeople in hygiene and safety precautions, arranging diets in the canteen for workers under medical care, and the keeping of appropriate records.

The *Health and Safety at Work Act 1974*, is designed to protect people at work and to prevent risks to the health and safety of the general public from working processes, such as the emission of dangerous or offensive substances into the air. The Act covers all working people—employers, employees, the self-employed—except domestic servants in private employment. Plant, systems of work, and premises have to be safe; staff have to be trained and supervised in safe ways of working; and designers and manufacturers have to ensure that their products are safe to use.

### Factory Conditions

To prevent sickness and accidents and to promote health and efficiency, the conditions under which people work have to be studied.

*Ventilation* should, as elsewhere, ensure the provision of fresh air without the production of draughts. About 1,000 cubic feet of fresh air should be provided per person per hour and kept in gentle motion. Where harmful dusts and gases are produced by the industrial processes a system of 'local exhaust ventilation' should suck them away from workpeople (see Fig. 25).

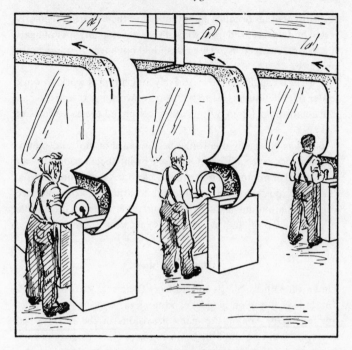

FIG. 25. *Local exhaust ventilation in a factory*

The *temperature* of a factory should be about 55° F (13° C) for heavy work, 60° F (16° C) for fairly active work, and 65° F (18° C) for light work. Protective clothing and goggles may have to be worn where heat production is extreme.

Good *lighting* is essential and should be provided by high, large windows (which should be kept clean), by tubular fluorescent lighting, and where fine work demands it local lighting without glare. Poor lighting is liable to produce poor work, depression and accidents.

*Noise* in excessive amount for long periods is fatiguing and psychologically disabling, and by permanently damaging the inner ear can produce irreparable deafness. The noise produced by a machine should be reduced as much as possible; workpeople exposed to excessive amounts of noise should wear protectors in the form of plugs or muffs and should have their hearing regularly tested and be removed from work if they develop any loss of hearing; people engaged in quiet work should not have to endure noisy processes.

*Fatigue* is usually due to excessively long hours of work, to work under poor conditions, or to bad ways of working. It leads to bad workmanship, a fall in output, absenteeism and excessive rates of sickness.

*Boredom* is usually due to the performance of dull and monotonous work especially when it is done by intelligent people. It can be avoided or minimized by a proper selection of personnel, music, changes in posture (e.g. from standing to sitting at work and vice versa), to ten-minute breaks for rest and refreshment in the middle of a work period, and by week-ends off and a summer holiday.

### Offices and Shops

Under the Offices, Shops and Railway Premises Act, 1963, which affects over 8 million people, conditions of work in these places are regulated. Among the many provisions of the Act are: (a) premises, furniture and fittings must be kept clean, (b) over-crowding is prohibited, (c) the temperature must be reasonable and a thermometer provided for each room, (d) ventilation and lighting must be adequate, (e) adequate sanitary conveniences, washing facilities, and drinking water must be provided, (f) facilities must be provided for storing and drying clothes, (g) seats must be provided where the job can be done sitting down, (h) work on dangerous machines is controlled, and (i) first aid facilities must be provided and placed in the care of a responsible and named person.

### Accidents

In some kinds of work, such as coalmining, the accident rate is high, largely because of the dangerous nature of the work. In other kinds of work, accidents are usually due to human factors, to a human mistake or act of carelessness. Every year in England and Wales nearly 1,000 people are killed by accidents at work, that is

3–4 every working day, and over 500,000 are so severely injured that they are off work for more than three days. Three out of four of these industrial accidents are due to: faulty methods of handling materials, falling, using machines dangerously, or being hit by a falling or moving object.

Accidents are particularly liable to occur when people are tired or bored. Too low a temperature in the factory makes people clumsy, too high a temperature makes them sleepy, and in both conditions accidents are particularly liable to happen. Young and inexperienced workpeople are particularly liable to accidents because they have not acquired the necessary skill or experience for a job; but, on the other hand, experienced people may become casualties by taking risks with machinery they know to be dangerous. About three-quarters of the number of accidents happen to about one-quarter of the people exposed to them, for reasons that are not very clear; such people are called accident-prone.

Accidents may be prevented by: (a) good factory conditions, (b) adequate precautionary measures against known dangers, e.g. the fencing in of moving parts, (c) not allowing people to work a dangerous machine without proper training and supervision, (d) not allowing any person to clean machinery in motion, and (e) taking adequate fire precautions.

### Selection of Personnel

An important aspect of industrial health is the selection of the right person for a job—putting a round peg in a round hole. In large industries this may be done by an industrial psychologist, in smaller industries by the personnel manager or manager. He should know intimately the job and what it demands. He will look for someone with:

(a) the right build, physical strength, eyesight and hearing;

(b) an appropriate degree of intelligence;

(c) the minimum standards for entry, e.g. the right technical training or examination passes;

(d) an aptitude for the job and the possession of any special skills required;

(e) the kind of disposition the job would suit.

People selected in this way are not likely to fail at a job, will be happier at it, will require less time for training, will have a higher rate of production, and will make fewer errors than people picked at random.

## Women in Industry

Many women are employed in industry. The work they do is less strenuous than that done by strong men, but many women are capable of doing heavy work without suffering ill effects. Menstruation seems to have little effect on working capacity. The accident rate of women is less than that of men. Women must not work in factories within one month of childbirth, and they are banned from working underground.

## Occupational Diseases

There are many kinds of occupational disease; some typical ones are described here.

**Blindness** in industrial workers is usually due to cataract (an opacity of the lens of the eye) produced by long exposure to high temperatures (e.g. in glass-workers) and infra-red waves (e.g. in tin-plate and sheet-metal workers).

**Deafness** is usually due to the constant repetition of loud noise, especially that produced by pneumatic and vibrating tools. It is common among weavers, boiler-makers and sheet-metal workers, who are all exposed to loud noise. The deafness is usually for a certain range of notes, and a workman may actually be able to hear better in a noisy workshop than in a quiet room.

**Vibration Effects.** Modern power-driven tools, vibrating two to three thousand times a minute, are liable to produce in the fingers of people using them the phenomena of Raynaud's disease. After several years of handling these tools, their fingers are liable to go white, bloodless and insensitive; cyanosis and gangrene may develop later. Among workpeople this condition is known as 'white fingers', 'dead fingers' or 'dead hand'.

**X-ray Injuries.** X-rays are used in many industrial processes, e.g. in the examination of metals, welded parts, cables, gas cylinders and golf balls. Workmen are unfortunately liable to treat with contempt a risk they cannot see. In consequence they may develop a dermatitis of exposed skin, which may lead to ulceration and carcinoma; the embryo in a pregnant woman may be affected; and in both sexes the genes in the sex-cells may develop abnormalities of structure. Any worker liable to be exposed to radiation should be warned of its dangers and carefully supervised. Adequate protection must be given by lead aprons, screens and windows, and the walls of all rooms in which X-ray apparatus is installed should be made impermeable by radiation.

**Heat Diseases.** Many people, such as stokers, foundry workers, furnacemen, glass-blowers and lime-kiln workers, are exposed to high temperatures in their work and may suffer in consequence. The three forms of heat disease are heat fatigue, heat cramp and heat exhaustion.

*Heat fatigue* is characterized by sweating, thirst, headache, irritability and emotional exhaustion. In temperate climates it is liable to occur in the summer months when there is an increase in atmospheric humidity and a diminution of the movement of air.

*Heat cramp* is characterized by severe muscular contraction, pain, exhaustion and sometimes albuminuria. It is due to a loss of chloride from the body by sweating, occurs usually during the second half of a shift, and can be relieved by drinking salt water.

*Heat exhaustion* is rare in temperate climates and usually occurs only in the tropics. It is a more severe condition than the other heat diseases and is characterized by prostration, nausea, vomiting, fever, visual disturbances and circulatory collapse.

**Caisson Disease.** A caisson is a steel or iron cylinder open at the bottom and used in underwater constructions. Water is kept out of the caisson by air being pumped in at a high pressure. This high pressure causes the blood of men working in a caisson to take up additional amounts of nitrogen; and if this pressure is too suddenly reduced bubbles of free nitrogen appear in the blood. The symptoms produced include severe pruritus, violent pains in the muscles (called by the workmen the 'bends', 'screws' or 'staggers'), nystagmus, blindness, cerebral lesions, and sometimes death from a cerebral haemorrhage. It can be prevented and treated by slow decompression of workmen in special chambers attached to the caisson; the longer the man has been exposed to pressure, the longer must be the period of decompression when he leaves the caisson.

**Miner's Nystagmus** is an oscillation of the eyeballs from side to side liable to occur in coal-miners. It may produce no symptoms and does not cause blindness, but it may cause night blindness and dancing of lights. Miners are liable to develop it about the age of forty after at least ten years' work at the coal-face. Its causation is obscure; it appears to be partly a physical and partly a psychological disability.

**Occupational Cramp** may be produced by the rapid repetition of fine movements and is liable to occur in writers, telegraphists, typists and musicians. It is characterized by spasm, tremor and weakness of the muscles of the hand and forearm. Anxiety is a common factor and tends to perpetuate the condition.

**Silicosis,** the commonest of the pneumoconioses or dust diseases, is due to the prolonged inhalation of fine particles of silica. Silica forms a large part of the earth's crust; and people particularly exposed to the dust are miners, tunnel cutters, stone-masons, sand-blasters, glass-makers, potters, people engaged in metallurgic processes, and people employed in the manufacture and use of abrasives.

Silicosis takes between five and twenty years to develop, the rate of its progress depending upon the number of particles of it in the air breathed in. The particles stick in the lungs, fibrous nodules form round them, a severe generalized fibrosis develops in the lungs, gross structural changes may be produced, and pulmonary tuberculosis often develops in a chronic form. The symptoms are cough and an increasing shortness of breath, and the diagnosis can be made on the occupational history and the characteristic X-ray findings.

The methods used to prevent this disease are improvements in general ventilation, special ventilation to remove dust, the damping down and removal of dust by sprays of water, and the wearing of protective devices over the nose and mouth.

**Asbestosis,** due to the inhalation of asbestos particles, is another form of pneumoconiosis, liable to occur in workmen making brake linings, clutch rings, millboard and asbestos tiles. The pathological signs and symptoms of the disease are similar to those of silicosis; it incapacitates more quickly, but is not so liable to produce pulmonary tuberculosis. The protective measures used are similar to those for silicosis.

**Industrial Dermatitis** is an inflammation of the skin produced by chemical substances, which may be dust, fumes or liquid, and by radiation. The symptoms are irritation, redness, papules and vesicles, which appear first on the hands, arms and other exposed parts of the body and later on other parts of the body; it closely resembles eczema and dermatitis of non-industrial origin.

It is common among engineers, workers in chemical industries, bread bakers and french polishers, and among the chemicals commonly responsible for its production are trinitrotoluene, mercury salts, chromic acid, alkalies, paraffin, turpentine, mineral oil, tar, formaldehyde, and some woods. It can be produced by exposure to X-rays, radioactive substances and actinic rays. Some people are more prone to get it than others, possibly as a result of constitutional factors such as an excessively dry or moist skin or of acquired factors such as previous attacks of dermatitis.

Prevention is by: (a) careful selection of workpeople and not employing people with a history of previous attacks of dermatitis or eczema in a job where they might be liable to develop industrial dermatitis; 'patch tests' on the skin may help to eliminate sensitive people; (b) the use of barrier creams (water-proof or oil-proof according to the nature of the chemical), gloves and other kinds of protective clothing; (c) regular inspection of workpeople for early signs of the disease; (d) the maintenance of a high standard of cleanliness with conveniently placed washing facilities where hands and arms can be washed after work (the degree of dermatitis bearing a relation to the duration and degree of contact of the chemical with the skin); and (e) arrangements for changing soiled clothing after work.

**Lead Poisoning.** Industrial lead poisoning is usually caused by the inhalation of particles of lead or lead salts or by taking food with unwashed hands. The trades with a lead hazard include painting, pottery manufacture, electric battery manufacture, and ship-breaking. Common symptoms and signs of lead poisoning are constipation, headache, anaemia, colic, dizziness, joint pains, wrist drop, and (in chronic cases) atherosclerosis and nephritis.

A high blood-level has been found in the children of lead workers, probably as a result of absorption of lead brought home on the worker's person, clothing or car; and there is a hazard to the health of children living in the neighbourhood of some lead works.

**Benzene Poisoning.** Benzene is used in dry-cleaning and in the rubber and explosives industries. Acute poisoning may produce severe effects, including mental excitement or coma. Chronic poisoning produces agranulocytosis (failure of the body to develop the granulocyte form of white blood cells), haemorrhages and death.

**Organic Phosphorus Poisoning.** Organic phosphorus compounds are used in horticulture and agriculture as pesticides. They can be absorbed through the lungs, bowels and skin, with the production of vomiting, abdominal pain, diarrhoea, twitching, difficulty in breathing, and death from coma or respiratory failure. Strict precautions to prevent absorption are taken during manufacture, packing and use, and care has to be taken that food is not contaminated when the pesticide is being transported from one place to another. A tractor driver engaged in spreading it should work inside a totally enclosed cabin.

# Chapter Eighteen

# RADIATION RISKS

The amount of radioactivity to which the human body is now exposed presents a new and major problem in hygiene and one that the modern nurse should have some knowledge of. In the last fifty years the amount of radioactivity has been enormously increased by the use of X-rays in diagnosis and treatment, by the use of radium in medicine, by the development of atomic energy, and by the explosion of nuclear weapons. This increase is of great importance because it may seriously affect both people alive today and unborn generations.

Atomic radiations are also called ionizing radiations. They may take the form of:

1. gamma rays given off by radioactive substances, and X-rays produced by special high-voltage equipment;
2. alpha and beta particles given off by radioactive isotopes.

All these have similar effects on living tissues.

The dose of ionizing radiations received by a person is expressed in 'rads'. A Geiger counter is an instrument for detecting the presence of radioactivity and measuring its amount.

Man has always been exposed to a small amount of radioactivity—by cosmic radiation from outer space (probably from the stars), by radiations off rocks and soil, and by radioactivity from his own body, which contains traces of radium absorbed over years and concentrated in his bones. The amount of radioactivity received from these sources is very small and amounts only to 0.1 to 0.15 rad a year, which does not do any harm.

But man has developed the following sources of radioactivity in amounts very much larger than those he is naturally exposed to:

*In Medicine:*
    X-rays—for diagnosis and treatment.

Radium—in the treatment of cancer.

Radioactive isotopes—for diagnosis and treatment.

*In Industry and Scientific Research*

Nuclear generating stations and their products.

X-rays—used in many industries.

Radioactive isotopes—used in many industries and laboratories.

*In Warfare:*

Nuclear weapons both at the time of the explosion and by producing a radioactive dust, which is gradually deposited over the earth.

*In Daily Life:*

Luminous paint—on watch and instrument dials, and X-ray machines—in shoe shops, may still be occasionally found.

Of all these sources of radioactivity the greatest increase is due to the use of X-rays for diagnosis.

The amount of radiation to which man is now exposed is capable of producing serious effects in the cells of his body. The cells particularly sensitive to radiation are those that grow quickly, such as:

the male and female sex cells

the cells of the blood

the cells of the mucous membranes of the stomach and small intestine

the cells of the skin (and also cancer cells).

The effects of radiation may be immediate, producing the disease called radiation sickness, or not apparent for several years. A single dose of 600 rads would be fatal to most people; a single dose of between 100 and 500 rads would produce symptoms varying in intensity with the dose received; and a single dose above 25 rads will produce abnormal changes in the blood. Exposure to doses of less than 1 rad a week over several years produces slight symptoms. Workers in hospital, research and industry should not be exposed to more than 0.3 rad in any one week, which is the maximum safe dose; few workers in Britain are exposed to this amount, modern techniques having made exposure of this size unnecessary, and the maximum permitted value will probably be reduced. If proper safety regulations are observed, there is no need to worry.

When diagnostic X-rays are taken, the patient will inevitably be exposed to radiation, and the radiologist, radiographer and nurse in the room will receive some unless they are adequately protected. The amount of radiation received by the patient varies with the part of the body being X-rayed, an X-ray of the chest exposing him to less than 1 rad and an X-ray of the pelvis to up to 10 rads. The dosage received by a person in this way is unlikely to affect him personally, but it is possible that it may affect the genes in his sex cells and so affect his descendants.

It is important that nurses working in wards where patients are receiving treatment by radium should not be exposed to radiation for dangerously long periods and should not have to spend in close proximity to the patients more time than is necessary to give adequate nursing attention. It is recommended that: (a) anaesthetics which have only a short recovery time should be used; (b) transport to the X-ray department should be avoided; (c) beds should be placed in such a position that nurses are not exposed to radiation while attending to other patients or engaged in other duties; and (d) mobile lead screens should be placed round the patient while nurses are in the neighbourhood.

X-ray shoe-fitting machines, once used in many shoe shops, give off radiations that are liable to affect customers and shop-assistants. These are now seldom found. In view of the dubious value of this method of fitting shoes and the possibility of multiple exposures, a nurse is advised not to make use of the machine.

## Clinical Effects of Radiation

### On Living People

*Radiation Sickness* is produced in people exposed to over 100 rads. Such an exposure may occur at the explosion of a nuclear bomb. If the person exposed is not killed, he will develop symptoms varying in severity with the dose of radiation received. The cells particularly affected are those of the blood, skin and mucous membrane of the alimentary tract. Antibody production may be stopped and the patient die of severe infection. If he lives he may in time develop cancer of the skin and internal organs, or cataract and may age prematurely.

*Leukaemia* may be produced by the therapeutic application of X-rays to the whole body.

*Radium needles* may produce degenerative changes in the fingers of surgeons or nurses who handle them.

**On the Unborn Child.** The effects on an unborn child vary with the age of the child and the amount of exposure. A large dose of X-rays, as might be used in the irradiation of the maternal pelvis for cancer, or of gamma rays from an atomic explosion, received within the first month of intra-uterine life would kill the child. Smaller doses received within the second or third month would interfere with the normal growth of the child and might produce mental retardation, physical abnormalities of the brain and spinal cord, congenital heart disease, cataract of the eye, and deformities of the skeleton. After three months the danger to the structural development of the child would not be so great, but the child would be likely to be small at birth and never to develop to normal stature.

**On Future Generations.** Small doses of radiation are likely to affect the sex cells of men and women. Within the sex cells are minute structures called genes, which are the factors deciding inheritance They are particularly sensitive to doses of radiation so small that they have no effect on the man or woman in whose genes the changes are taking place. Changes in genes are called mutations and are liable to have serious effects on the development of future children.

**What Can a Nurse Do?** There are some things a nurse can do to reduce the amount of radiation received by her and her patients. She should:

1. Strictly observe all safety instructions in any place where X-rays are taken or radioactive material used.

2. Not handle radium needles with her fingers, but use the proper forceps.

3. Not press for X-rays, especially for women who may be pregnant.

4. Not have her feet examined by X-ray machines in shoe shops.

5. Not wear a watch with a luminous dial; or if she does wear one, not wear it when she is asleep and liable to irradiate her ovaries with it.

6. Study *The Safe Use of Ionising Radiations* (H.M. Stationery Office).

## Micro-waves

Micro-waves are used in catering and domestic ovens, industrial heating, radio-navigation, etc. Exposure can produce cataracts, corneal opacities, degeneration of the testes and haemorrhagic disorder: the most vulnerable part is the eye. A maximum permissible safety level for human exposure has been fixed. Apparatus should be so designed with appropriate screening that the danger level is not exceeded.

# Chapter Nineteen

# THE NURSE'S HEALTH

A nurse should come physically fit to her training and must endeavour to keep herself fit. Much of the work she does will be physically hard; she will have to stand for long periods and walk far, almost all her work will be done indoors, much of it will be mentally trying. When she comes off duty she may feel too tired and listless to eat a good meal or to take some exercise in the open air. But all the time she must remember to apply to herself the basic principles of hygiene and in spite of all difficulties be to her patients a shining example of positive health.

**Occupational Health Service.** The Occupational Health Service of a hospital exists to maintain at a high level the health of all staff in the hospital. It is staffed by a doctor and nurses who have taken a course in occupational health.

It is principally responsible for: the medical examination of certain staff (medical, nursing, catering, laundry) on joining the service; the health education of staff; the immunization of staff against communicable disease; X-ray of chests of staff (usually every 3 years, more frequently of those working in high-risk areas); the study and improvement of working conditions; receiving and acting on reports of accidents to staff; rehabilitation of staff after illness or accident; keeping medical records of staff.

**Tests and Inoculations.** The particularly dangerous communicable diseases that she may find herself exposed to, wherever she is nursing, are:

tuberculosis, especially the pulmonary variety
typhoid and paratyphoid fevers
smallpox

She may have been immunized against these in childhood, and she should know what she has been immunized against and when.

She should be willing to have any further immunization considered necessary.

Her chest will be X-rayed for evidence of pulmonary tuberculosis and a tuberculin test will be done. If her tuberculin test is negative, she should be willing to be immunized with BCG vaccine.

**On Duty.** A nurse should not come on duty if she feels ill, has a cold or running nose, has septic spots on her skin or has diarrhoea, but should report herself sick.

She should have a hot bath daily. It will refresh her, keep her skin clean and healthy, and make her smell pleasant to the patients with whom she is in close contact.

She should be scrupulously careful to keep her hands and nails clean, and to wash them before and after handling patients, after going to the lavatory, before handling food, before meals and on leaving the ward.

She should be immaculate in her appearance and clothing. Her clothing should be adequate and warm. She must remember that nylons and other artificial fabrics must not be worn in an operating theatre because the friction of nylon against nylon may produce enough static electricity to spark off an explosion of ether vapour.

If she is on duty all day, she should change her shoes and stockings during the day and wear another pair of each. On coming off duty she should rest her feet by changing her shoes.

**Off Duty.** A nurse should take reasonable amounts of recreation and exercise; but she should not try to do too much when she is tired and she should not play games beyond the point of fatigue. Every day she ought to have at least a walk in the open air. This is particularly applicable to nurses who live in a Nurses' Hostel close to the hospital in which they work and whose only outdoor exercise might become no more than a rush from one to the other. In addition to taking outdoor exercise or playing games, a nurse may choose to join a Keep-Fit class and so keep her body and limbs supple.

If a nurse likes to go out dancing or to the cinema, it is inadvisable for her to have more than one late night in a fortnight and she must not have two late nights in succession. A nurse should aim at always being at her best. She cannot be a good nurse if she is tired and dull; she cannot then work well, will cease to be a pleasure and a stimulus to her patients, and will become more liable to make mistakes.

She should try to get eight hours' sound sleep every night in a well-ventilated bedroom.

It is very important that she should eat good meals of the basic foods. When she feels too tired to eat she should try to eat a small meal rather than nothing at all.

She should weigh herself once a month, stripped or in the same weight of clothes. She should compare her weight with the scale for her age and build. A young nurse should aim at keeping her weight a few pounds above the average; a nurse over forty should aim at keeping hers at the average. Slight gains or losses in weight may be corrected easily by slight changes in diet. It is much easier to make these slight adjustments than to correct large gains or losses.

A persistent loss of weight should be reported.

**Night Duty** is a particularly trying time for a nurse because the whole daily pattern of her life has to be changed. As a result of this change she may get little sleep, lose her appetite, and develop feelings of weariness and inertia. To fall asleep by day may be very difficult for her, and what sleep she gets may be short and broken. She will have to find out for herself whether she sleeps better just after coming off duty or later in the day. Even though she does not have a good appetite she should try to eat good meals. Every day she should get some exercise in the open air.

**Study.** Some of the nurse's time is necessarily spent in studying for examinations. Except for her spells of night duty, when she should not try to study at all (for the amount she would retain would be slight or nil), she should work so steadily throughout her training that she has no need to cram for long hours just before her examinations.

# Chapter Twenty

# COMMUNITY HEALTH

An Area Health Authority of the National Health Service is responsible for many services, including:

    health visiting
    domiciliary midwifery
    care of mothers and young children
    dental care of mothers and young children
    family planning
    environmental health in liaison with local authorities and water
    authorities
    health education
    control of communicable diseases
    immunization against communicable diseases
    chiropody
    ambulance service
    supervision of private nursing homes
Its staff will include community physicians, health visitors, domiciliary midwives.

A *local authority* (not a health authority) is responsible for:
social services, care of unmarried mothers and their children, supervision of child minders, day nurseries and play groups, and domestic help for those in need of it and also for many aspects of environmental health.

## Area Health Authority Clinics

An Area Health Authority maintains clinics for the benefit of people living in its area and staffs them with appropriate doctors, nurses, specialists and supporting staff. The kinds of clinic provided vary from authority to authority, but among them are likely to be the following:

**Antenatal Clinic.** An antenatal clinic is responsible for: examination of expectant women, in co-operation with the hospital or family doctor; taking of specimens for laboratory investigations; parenthood classes for both parents; relaxation classes; health education of pregnant women.

**Postnatal Clinic.** A postnatal clinic is responsible for the examination of mother and child about six weeks after delivery if this is not done at a hospital or by the family doctor.

**Family Planning Clinic.** A family planning clinic advises on birth-control, subfertility and marital problems. For this work the health authority may call upon the services of a branch of the Family Planning Association.

**Clinic for Retired People.** A clinic for retired people may be associated with a Darby and Joan club and conducted on the same premises. Retired people are invited to attend for: medical examination, testing of sight and hearing, dental examination, urine examination, and examination of blood, especially for haemoglobin, sugar and urea levels.

**The Care of Old People.** Many more people are now living into old age, and this increase in their numbers increases the social and medical problems they produce. Although some people retain health, vigour and mental alertness into old age, many others, as a result of genetic and environmental factors, become senile and in consequence require much help. The especial troubles of old age are loneliness, unwantedness, poverty, bad housing conditions, ill health, physical weakness, undernutrition, anxiety and mental deterioration. Old people who continue to work and take responsibility decline less than those who have nothing to do and for whom life is merely 'waiting for the end', and it is important that old people should feel wanted and do work within their capacity for as long as possible.

Old people may be lonely because they are widowed, because they have moved from their home to a new home at the seaside, because their children have gone to live elsewhere, and their friends and contemporaries have died or themselves become infirm and unable to visit them. Old people may cling to their old home, however unsuitable it may be for them to live in. Because of ignorance, poverty or apathy their diet is often inadequate, especially in proteins and vitamins; old widowers tend to live on food that requires little preparation or cooking; and physical weakness and mental confusion are likely to be produced. Their sight, hearing and sense of smell may decline, their feet be crippled by corns, and their muscular co-ordination become impaired. They are particularly liable to accidents by falling. Senile or arteriosclerotic dementia may add to their troubles and the difficulty of looking after them.

Help is provided by the Local Authority, the National Health Service and voluntary organizations.

Home helps can be provided to do the old person's housework. The district nurse will assist with bathing, giving injections or other treatment, and doing dressings. The Local Authority can arrange for the washing of the clothes and bedclothes of incontinent people and for the loan of equipment such as bedpans and waterproof sheets. A Health Visitor spends much of her time looking after old people and especially those who live alone. She should help to prepare old people for retirement and encourage and train their relatives to look after them. She will be in a position to assess the need of an old person for social and medical assistance and should know how it can be provided. A 'Meals on Wheels' service provides one good meal a day. Where there is financial hardship the retirement pension can be supplemented by special allowances. Old people should be encouraged to join an Old Folks' Club, where they will find companionship, meals, games and outings.

The residential accommodation provided by the Local Authority or by voluntary organizations includes small houses or ground-floor flats for old people and sometimes a resident warden to look after them, homes in which old people can have their own furniture, and homes of senile people not able to look after themselves or their belongings. The National Health Service is responsible for providing hospital accommodation for old people who need it. This may take the form of special geriatric units or day hospitals, in which they are looked after by day and from which they go home at night to be looked after by their own people.

Geriatric physicians are available for consultation and advice on the care and treatment of the old.

**Sexually-Transmitted Diseases.** Sexually-transmitted diseases, of which the most important are syphilis and gonorrhoea, present major medical and social problems.

Special clinics are provided by the Health Service. These clinics are open at convenient times, such as the afternoon or evening, with separate times for men and women, and provisions are made to avoid publicity. To encourage people to come for treatment, these diseases are not notifiable, and all information obtained from patients is strictly confidential. An infected person is asked to persuade any sexual partner to come to the clinic for investigation or to allow a Health Visitor or Social Worker to approach him or her. Defaulters, i.e. patients who have started but not completed a course of treatment, may have to be traced and persuaded to return for the full course.

**Mental Disorders.** Provisions for mentally disordered people are the responsibility of both Local Authorities and the Health Service. A Local Authority has to provide educational services for mentally handicapped children, both in and out of hospital, and to provide hostels and training centres for adults. Hospital services are a part of the Health Service and are provided both in special wards and clinics in general hospitals or in special psychiatric hospitals. Most patients enter them 'informally' as they would a medical or surgical ward, but a few have to be compulsorily detained in accordance with the provisions of the Mental Health Act 1959. The patient at home will be assisted by a Social Worker or by a hospital-based Community Nurse.

### The Health Visitor

*Employment.* Health visitors are employed by Area Health Authorities.

*Qualifications*

(a) State registration in nursing and

(b) SCM or Part I midwifery or obstetric nurse training as part of the training for SRN and

(c) Health visitor training. Health visitor training is for one year, at a technical college or university, five 'O' levels being usually required before acceptance for training.

*Aims.* The principal aim of the health visitor is the promotion of health, physical, mental and social, of all age-groups, in the district she is responsible for. Health visitors work in the homes of patients, in clinics, health centres, general practitioner surgeries, and hospitals. The health visitor may hold a joint appointment as health visitor/school nurse.

**Responsibilities**

(a) *Children.* The birth of any baby in the district assigned to her is notified to the health visitor and she takes over from the midwife about the tenth day after birth. The health visitor continues to visit the home according to her assessment of the needs of mother and child.

She gives advice to mothers on upbringing, diet and health, on times for immunizations, and on the prevention of accidents in the home.

She organizes parentcraft classes, for fathers as well as for mothers, and gives advice on family planning. She studies the developing child, keeps records of his progress, physical, intellectual, emotional, and endeavours to detect any abnormality, e.g. mental retardation, any defect of hearing, any defect of vision, epilepsy, spasticity.

She studies home conditions and is alert for any evidence of neglect or ill-treatment of the child, such as baby-battering.

When she considers it necessary, she advises the parents to take the child to their doctor or to an appropriate clinic, and she can put them into touch with an official or voluntary organizations.

(b) *Care of old people.* Much of the time of a health visitor is spent in looking after old people and especially those who live alone. She should prepare people for retirement and old age, and should encourage and train relatives to look after them. She is in a position to assess the need of an old person for social and medical assistance, and should know how it can be provided.

(c) *Patients with communicable diseases.* The health visitor is a member of the team engaged in the prevention of communicable diseases. Part of her work may be in an immunization clinic, and she is concerned in the instruction of parents in the appropriate times for their children to be immunized. She helps to trace contacts.

The health visitor visits the homes of people notified as suffering from tuberculosis. She advises the patient and his relatives how to prevent the spread of infection, on the importance of continuing drug treatment, and how to try to cope with domestic and financial difficulties that arise. She arranges for contacts to be X-rayed or .uberculin-tested.

### The Domiciliary Midwife

*Employment.* The domiciliary midwife is employed by an Area Health Authority.

*Qualifications.* State Certified Midwife.

**Responsibilities.** The duties of the domiciliary midwife are the ante-natal care, delivery and postnatal care of those mothers who decide to have their babies born at home. She works in cooperation with general-practitioner obstetricians and may work in an attachment scheme with a group of general practitioners.

*Antenatal care.* The midwife:

   participates in the antenatal care of women booked for delivery at home, and often for those booked for delivery at hospital;

   advises on the suitability of the home for delivery or for early discharge from hospital;

   conducts parenthood classes for mothers and fathers·

   advises on claiming maternity benefits;

   arranges with the social services for the provision of home helps, etc.;

   tries to trace defaulters from antenatal clinics.

*Delivery.* The midwife conducts deliveries at home or in general practitioner units in hospital.

*Postnatal care.* The midwife cares for mother and child for ten days after delivery, arranges for the attendance of the mother for postnatal examination, and hands over mother and child to the health visitor about the tenth day after delivery.

## The Environmental Health Officer

Environmental health officers are employed by Local Authorities in the promotion of environmental health. Their work includes:

the inspection of food for sale;

the inspection of dairies and milk-pasteurization plants;

water sampling;

the supervision of slaughterhouses and the inspection of meat;

the inspection of premises where 'offensive trades' are carried out;

the inspection of houses for sanitary and other defects;

the disinfection and disinfestation of bedding, clothes and houses;

the destruction of vermin;

smoke abatement;

noise abatement;

the control of communicable diseases by advice and by tracing contacts;

the inspection of offices for toilet facilities, cleanliness and lighting;

the investigation of complaints involving community health.

The environmental health officer tries to see that laws are enforced and good health standards maintained; and he does this not so much by threatening or taking legal action as by persuading personnel at all levels to do what should be done to maintain a high standard of environmental health.

## School Health Service

The school health service is directed by the Area Health Authority.

Its purpose is the promotion of health and the detection of handicaps and disease in school children. The service is provided for all schools maintained by the Education Authority and can be provided by arrangement for children in private schools.

## Staff

1. *Medical.* The *principal school medical officer* is usually the local principal community physician. The medical staff carry out medical examinations.

A *child psychiatrist* sees and treats children referred to him with psychiatric disorders.

An *anaesthetist* is provided for dental surgery requiring an anaesthetic.

2. *Nursing.* A joint appointment of health visitor/school nurse is commonly held. The nurse must have the qualifications of a health visitor. She is assisted by state registered and state enrolled nurses and by nursing assistants.

3. *Dental.* The *school dental officer* and his supporting staff.

4. *Other Specialists*

Educational psychologist

Social worker

Speech therapist

Remedial gymnast

Chiropodist

**Medical Examinations.** Medical examinations are carried out three times during a child's school life: during the first school year, at about 11 years old, and during the last school year. An additional *eye examination* may be carried out at about 8 years.

Examinations at other times can be requested by a parent, teacher, school nurse or a doctor.

Particular attention is paid to:

the detection of defective vision or hearing;

nutrition;

educational subnormality;

physical handicaps, e.g. heart disease, epilepsy, spasticity, muscular dystrophy;

speech handicaps;

emotional disturbances.

Should treatment be required, the child is referred to his own doctor, to a hospital or to an appropriate clinic maintained by the Area Health Authority.

*School Nurse.* The work of the school nurse is mainly in:
attending medical examination and immunization clinics;
testing sight and hearing;
examination of children for head infestation, cleanliness, and any evidence of parental neglect or brutality;
assisting in measures to prevent the spread of communicable diseases in the school;
giving health education to children;
visiting homes and liaising between school, clinic and home in any matter affecting the child's health.

### District Nursing Service

The district nursing service carries out those forms of nursing care which can be carried out in the home and do not require the facilities of a hospital. Its staff consists of:

(a) a team composed of a district nursing sister or male nurse (SRN with district training) and a district auxiliary or attendant (with inservice training), or

(b) a State Registered Nurse, working on her own.

The members of the district nursing service are employed by the Area Health Authority. A district nursing sister may act as liaison officer between hospital and home. The team may be attached to a group of general practitioners.

The work includes:
bathing, attention to pressure points, cleaning the mouth;
injections, catheterization, giving enemas, bandaging, removal of sutures;
recording pulse, respiration, temperature, blood pressure;
obtaining and forwarding specimens for laboratory investigation;
counselling the patient and his relatives;
instruction of relatives in the custody and administration of

drugs, and in the disposal of unwanted drugs, soiled dressings and excreta;
putting the patient in touch with appropriate social services.

**Ambulance Service.** One of the functions of an Area Health Authority is to provide an ambulance service. Such a service is used for accidents and emergencies, for expectant mothers, for discharges from hospital, for transfer from one hospital to another, for taking patients to lectures and demonstrations, and for moving special medical equipment. When a long journey has to be undertaken, arrangements are made with British Rail for the transport of a stretcher case in a special compartment on a train.

## Social Service Department

The work of the Social Service Department of a local authority is carried out by social workers. The social workers may be employed in the community or attached to a hospital. There should be a close co-operation between nurses, doctors and social workers because much of their work overlaps and they are often concerned in assisting the same people.

The work of a Social Service Department embraces the following.

**Disabled Persons.** The department has the duty laid upon it to seek out disabled persons and to provide them with appropriate care and assistance.

**Children.** The department is responsible for:
the supervision of day nurseries, child minders and play groups;
the provision of residential nurseries;
the provision of facilities for the unmarried mother and her child;
the provision of facilities and advice for problem families;
the inspection of private nurseries and foster homes

**Mentally Ill and Mentally Handicapped Persons.** The department is responsible for: the provision of hostels, training centres and sheltered workshops; the support and supervision of patient and family.

**The Aged and Physically Handicapped.** The department is responsible for the support of old and handicapped people in their homes, e.g. by the provision of home helps to do the housework, cooking and shopping; by providing meals on wheels; by friendly visits; by carrying out alterations in the house such as the provision of rails and ramps, alterations in the kitchen and bathroom to enable the person to stay at home and carry out ordinary activities.

The social services department is also responsible for the provision of accommodation (this is called Part III accommodation, after the part of the Act of Parliament authorizing it); accommodation in nursing homes, special accommodation for the handicapped; accommodation in private homes.

The department also provides outings, holidays and clubs with social and occupational facilities.

**Homeless.** The department is responsible for the welfare of the homeless and the provision of temporary accommodation.

A Social Service Department may make charges for some of its provisions according to the means of the person assisted. It works in collaboration with appropriate voluntary organizations, to whom it can give financial aid.

# Chapter Twenty-one

# WORLD HEALTH

For the last hundred years various organizations have been engaged in establishing international codes of health. At first these organizations were engaged in studying and trying to control the major communicable diseases then so prevalent in epidemic form—diseases such as cholera, smallpox, yellow fever, plague and typhus. In 1923 the League of Nations established its Health Organization, which, as well as studying the major communicable diseases, turned its attention to such subjects as nutrition, cancer, malaria and the establishment of international biological standards.

In 1948 the World Health Organization (WHO) was established by the United Nations Organization (UNO). The principles upon which the WHO was to act were declared to be these:

'Health is a state of complete physical, mental and social well-being and not merely the absence of disease and infirmity.

'The enjoyment of the highest attainable standard of health is one of the fundamental rights of every human being without distinction of race, religion, political belief, economic or social condition.

'The health of all people is fundamental to the attainment of peace and security and is dependent upon the fullest co-operation of individuals and states.

'The achievement of any state in the promotion and protection of health is of value to all.

'Unequal development in different countries in the promotion of health and control of disease, especially communicable disease, is a common danger.

'Healthy development of the child is of basic importance; the ability to live harmoniously in a changing total environment is essential to such development.

'The extension to all peoples of the benefits of medical, psychological and related knowledge is essential to the fullest attainment of health.

'Informed opinion and active co-operation on the part of the public are of the utmost importance in the improvement of the health of the people.

'Governments have a responsibility for the health of their peoples which can be filled only by the provision of adequate health and social measures.'

The World Health Assembly is composed of delegates representing the member states of the WHO. It holds an annual meeting and special sessions at which problems of world health are discussed. It has an Executive Board and many Expert Committees on such subjects as Maternity and Child Welfare, Tuberculosis, Malaria, Venereal Disease, Quarantine, Atomic Energy. It has six Regional Organizations, covering the whole world, with Regional Headquarters at Copenhagen, Washington, Alexandria, Brazzaville, New Delhi and Manila.

**The Scope of WHO Activities** is intended to include all aspects of international health. Much of its work is advisory and instructional. It investigates problems of health and disease, but it has neither the funds nor the personnel to carry out what it considers advisable, and individual countries who have come to it for advice are expected to carry out the necessary health measures by their own efforts. Among the conditions and problems to which attention is given are:

1. The establishment of international health regulations for all forms of travel, in order to prevent the spread of infection from one country to another.

2. The study of the epidemics of communicable disease; daily information is given to member countries by radiotelegraphy from Geneva.

3. Large-scale attacks on disease-spreading insects, such as the mosquito that spreads malaria.

4. Housing and sanitation, especially in backward countries.

5. The training and effective use of nurses and midwives; the inclusion of nurses in demonstration teams going to

backward countries; conferences and study groups on nursing problems.

6. The establishment of better health services for women and children, especially for pregnant women, babies and handicapped children.

7. The establishment of better mental health services.

8. The reduction of tuberculosis by the mass vaccination of children and young people with BCG vaccine.

9. The prevention, control and cure of serious tropical diseases such as leprosy, yaws, trachoma and bilharziasis.

10. The development of peaceful uses of atomic energy in new methods of diagnosis and treatment; protection against radiation; the safe disposal of radioactive waste.

11. The standardization of drugs.

12. The control of addiction-producing drugs.

13. The improvement and standardization of health statistics.

14. The maintenance of library and reference services.

15. Technical education and training, by the award of fellow-ships to doctors, nurses and other health workers in order that they may study at special centres and in other countries, and by the free spread of the latest and best medical knowledge.

16. The health education of the public, especially in maternal and child welfare, mental health and nutrition.

17. The sending of international aid to countries stricken by disaster, such as an earthquake.

**Association with Other Organizations.** The WHO recognizes that the promotion of health is not entirely a medical and nursing problem, to be solved by doctors and nurses, and that it is just as much a social, political, economic, scientific and educational problem. Poverty, unrest, war, civil strife, unemployment, sloth, ignorance and superstition are major causes of the spread and persistence of ill health and disease. Accordingly in many of its activities WHO works in collaboration with other international organizations, such as:

UNESCO—the United Nations Educational, Scientific and Cultural Organization, which is especially concerned with the spread of education and science throughout the world (except medicine and health, which are the province of WHO).

UNICEF—the United Nations International Children's Emergency Fund, which is concerned with the health of children, their nutrition, and the conditions under which they live.

FAO—the Food and Agricultural Organization, which is concerned with nutrition, rural hygiene, and human diseases originating in animals.

ILO—the International Labour Organization, which is concerned with the health of workers, conditions of work, the health of seamen and the conditions under which they work and live, and the study of social and insurance schemes in various countries.

By the efforts of all these organizations acting in co-operation with WHO all over the world and particularly in the underdeveloped countries, disease is prevented and health vigorously promoted.

**Council of Europe.** Many European countries (including Britain) belong to the Council of Europe, whose headquarters are at Strasbourg. The improvement of public health and social services in Europe is one of the aims of the Council.

The co-ordination of medical services throughout Europe and the publication of a European Pharmacopoeia are at present being considered by the European Public Health Committee of this Council.

**International travel.** Sea and Air Port Health Authorities are concerned with the health and threats to health (particularly by communicable diseases not common in Britain, such as cholera) of people entering Britain. The size of the problem may be assessed by the large numbers concerned, over 20 million people passing through Heathrow Airport in 1973. Of these 20 million the staff of the health control unit saw nearly 1 million, medically examined over 47,000, and vaccinated 22,000 against smallpox, cholera or yellow fever.

# INDEX